Hip and Knee Replacement

W · W · NORTON & COMPANY · NEW YORK · LONDON

RYLE MILLER, JR.

GEOFFREY McCULLEN, M. D.

Hip and Knee Replacement

A PATIENT'S GUIDE

Drawings by Dolly Miller

First Edition

The text of this book is composed in Palatino with the display set in Peignot and Kaufman Script. Composition and manufacturing by The Maple-Vail Book Manufacturing Group. Book design by Marjorie J. Flock.

Library of Congress Cataloging-in-Publication Data

Miller, Ryle L.
  Hip and knee replacement : a patient's guide / Ryle Miller, Jr., and
    Geoffrey McCullen ; drawings by Dolly Miller.
      p.   cm.
  Includes index.
  ISBN 0-393-03834-3
  1. Total hip replacement—Popular works. 2. Total knee
  replacement—Popular works. I. McCullen, Geoffrey. II. Title.
  RD549.M36   1996
  617.5'810592—dc20   95-30196

W. W. Norton & Company, Inc., 500 Fifth Avenue, New York, N.Y. 10110
http://web.wwnorton.com
W. W. Norton & Company Ltd., 10 Coptic Street, London WC1A 1PU

1 2 3 4 5 6 7 8 9 0

CONTENTS

FIGURES

A Personal Prologue

THE FIRST HINT that my hips and knees would become the major preoccupation in my life came in 1971, when I was forty-eight years old, on vacation in France. My wife, Dolly, and I had planned our whole three-week vacation, down to every meal. We were touring the prehistoric caves in the Dordogne in southwestern France, staying in the Hôtel Cro-Magnon in Les Eyzies-de-Tayac, which we had chosen because it had a one-star restaurant in the *Guide Michelin*. We had lived in France for six years during the 1950s, when I had worked there as an engineer, and we had traveled extensively, using the *Michelin* guides. Now, after twelve years, we were going back for a visit with less money than we had before, but we hoped to make up for that with our knowledge.

Up until we reached the Cro-Magnon, things had gone according to prediction. We had stayed at a lovely hotel in Paris, called the Saxe Résidence, then taken a luxury train,

Le Mistral, to Nice, where we had rented a car, which we would drive back to Paris, touring the Dordogne along the way. In that way, our vacation was divided into three phases, an initial three days in Paris, the driving tour, and a final week in Paris. When I gave our list of reservations to the concierge at the Saxe Résidence, asking him to telephone each to confirm, he turned to the hotel's desk clerk and said: "Here are people who know how to travel."

Much to our disappointment, however, I seemed to be losing my zest for rich foods, until I not only lacked an appetite but could not eat. Then on the last day of our stay at the Cro-Magnon, I found myself so full of muscular pains and so sluggish that I could not go out to enjoy a beautiful sunset with Dolly, and I spent the evening in our room, while she went out by herself. Fortunately, I recovered during the drive back to Paris, and put the experience out of mind.

However, when we got back to New York, I experienced similar attacks but with more pain, until I ended up spending an entire weekend lying on my side facing the back of the sofa, and eventually missed some days at work. This was a new experience for me. I took the problem to our physician, Dr. Ira Laufer, who examined me and took blood tests, which confirmed the existence of pain as a general inflammation. When the attacks persisted, he had me admitted to New York University Hospital for two weeks of tests. He had been chief resident at NYU Hospital, and was proud of the renowned specialists who were available there.

Almost every second day of my two-week stay, a different doctor would appear in our four-bed ward room, identify me by the chart on the foot of my bed, and proceed to examine me. I could gauge the prestige of the physician examining me by the actions of the resident doctors on duty. Sometimes the examining doctor was barely gone when two or three of the resident doctors, who had been unobtrusively occupied elsewhere in the room, would converge on my chart in order to see what had been written there. Then later one or another of them would appear with an instrument bag and ask me to let him or her examine me again. Thus I was examined and reexamined. But there was no positive identification of my sickness, other than the confirmation that I was experiencing pain.

Fortunately for me, that mysterious pain had already been the subject of widespread medical research, and during the same period, of the early 1970s, the world medical profession was learning to accept a new design for artificial hip joints, which had been developed by Sir John Charnley, at the Wrightington Hospital in Lancashire, England. This design established that a hardened metal ball fitted to a metal extension of the thighbone would function satisfactorily in a ball-and-socket joint when the socket was made of ultra-high-density polyethylene, a hardened version of the same plastic that is used for coffee-can covers. The metal extension and the socket were held in place by dental cement, which is the acrylic resin polymethyl methacrylate. Experience with this artificial hip showed that 90% of the people who received it were rid of practically all pain and 80% recovered most of their joint motion. Although I knew nothing about them, those statistics were to become vitally important to the quality of my life.

In New York, meanwhile, Dr. Laufer referred me to the clinic at NYU Hospital of Dr. Thomas Kantor, a nationally known rheumatologist. When I first walked into that crowded clinic and saw his other patients I was embarrassed to be taking up his time. In the large waiting room, whose low ceiling seemed to make it even more crowded, there were people with canes, crutches, walkers, and wheelchairs. The most remarkable thing about them was a uniform facial expression showing a determined cheerfulness through pain. But Dr. Kantor soon had me enrolled in several of the latest treatments for my disease, which he diagnosed as rheumatism.

Dr. Laufer called my disease polymyositis, meaning inflamed muscles, because my blood tests did not give the specific indication for rheumatism, and polymyositis is effectively the same as rheumatism, i.e., a general inflammation of the muscles and tendons serving the joints. Then my knees began to swell, and Dr. Kantor began treating them with injections. Finally, one day Dr. Laufer told me that Dr. Kantor had identified arthritis, which is defined as an inflammation of the joints, so I was finally diagnosed as having rheumatoid arthritis.

Dr. Laufer and Dr. Kantor agreed to recommend entering me in a program of gold injections. Although it is not understood why or how gold injections combat arthritis, Dr. Kantor had statistical evidence to make him enthusiastic over their potential for me. The only trouble was that gold injections had to be administered once a week for nearly a year, during which I would need monitoring for both the effect on my rheumatoid arthritis and possible poisoning. I agreed, and we started the program, first at Dr. Kantor's clinic, and after a month, with Dr. Laufer. Also, in order to help the effect of the gold, we began with a series of cortisone pills, at 5 milligrams a day of prednisone, which would be phased out as the gold took effect.

The cortisone immediately brought a complete relief from my symptoms, and after about nine months, the gold injections brought about a remission. This was my first relief from pestering pains, general fatigue, and morning stiffness, which had become so ever-present that I was unaware not only of the symptoms but also of my reaction to them. I learned that my facial expressions were revealing my pains when, on the way to work one morning, I found a woman barring my way as I hurried against a yellow streetlight. "Take it easy, honey," she said, grinning. "You'll make it."

The remission achieved through the treatments with cortisone and gold gave me the confidence to begin planning a move to Vermont. Inspired by our love for the woods, Dolly and I had in 1970 bought a hundred acres of woodland between Lake Willoughby and Crystal Lake in Vermont's northeast lakes region, where we went for our vacations, staying at cabins on a farm overlooking Lake Willoughby. I had been trying to write fiction, and in order to develop writing skills had abandoned my successful engineering career for a job as a technical reporter on a weekly news magazine.

On early vacations I had been content to pass the weeks writing. But as the rejection slips piled up, I was forced to accept that I would never achieve my ambition of becoming a novelist, and I came to feel restless during those Vermont vacations, particularly when the farmer from whom we rented our cabin often completed a construction project that yielded something substantial, like a new cabin or a porch to his house, during the time of our stay, whereas I had nothing to show for our time but some pieces of paper. Dolly was also experiencing dissatisfaction. She had been trying to establish herself as an artist, and went regularly to the Art Students League in Manhattan. Although she had lots of recognition from other artists, she lacked the commercial sense that facilitates becoming established as a painter.

We had found that, living in metropolitan New York, we needed regular breaks from the city. We shared a tendency to seek out woods for our recreation. Although we had learned about Harriman Interstate Park (40,000 acres of woodland) and often went there for weekend hikes, we had felt we needed something more for our vacations. We had been attracted to Vermont's rural woodlands, where the Eastern Continental Divide separates the rivers flowing into the Connecticut from those flowing into the St. Lawrence; and we had become regular vacationers at Lake Willoughby.

At the time we began to make plans for a move to Vermont, the Charnley concept of a low-friction ball-and-socket joint had become established, and progress in the dynamic field of joint fabrication was advancing along two paths of research toward making the substitute joints longer-lasting. One path was to improve cement fixation by reducing the cement's viscosity and porosity and by pressurizing it. The other exploited the growth properties of living human bone by using beaded porous surfaces on metals like titanium that would encourage the bone to grow fast to the implanted metal part, eliminating the use of cement entirely.

Also, improved artificial knee joints were being designed according to concepts developed by Dr. Frank Gunston, of Winnepeg, Canada, who had worked with Charnley in England. Taking advantage of the low friction of metal on plastic, Gunston designed a fabricated knee joint that put two hardened-metal rockers into grooves in a high-density polyethylene plastic plate. By July 1978, when Dolly and I packed our belongings into a rented truck and moved to Vermont, the designs of artificial knees had also evolved two schools, depending on whether or not the artificial knee retained certain ligaments that connect the thighbone to the shinbone.

We arrived in Vermont with $4,000 in the bank and no source of income other than a 20% veteran's disability pension for a wound received in World War II. Right away, we were much too busy preparing for our first winter to think about Dr. Laufer, my gold shots, or even my rheumatism. With the failure to follow up with the gold shots, the remission of my rheumatism and arthritis wore off; and all the old familiar symptoms of morning stiffness, fatigue, and aching muscles came flooding through my body.

But their effects were different from those I had experienced in New York. Whereas I had merely felt inconvenienced and uncomfortable when confronted by threatening traffic while walking the streets of Manhattan, I now felt actually inadequate, for I had to build a house. As I tried to master the tools and techniques, the old feelings of anxiety were replaced by irritation and frustration. I grew angry at things. When I drove a nail with an aching arm and wrist, the nail seemed to bend of its own accord. When I strained to hold a plank in place with one hand while driving a nail to fasten it there, the plank seemed to take on an independent weight and to refuse to fit where I had just successfully tried it. The hammer holster on my belt seemed to travel around behind me, in order to evade the hammer I wanted to hang there. Poor Dolly, when she was compelled to work with me, wished aloud that I were not so irritable. But I usually worked alone, and with no one to overhear me, began to curse the inanimate objects I worked with. The more extravagant curses gave me some satisfaction, because of their shock value for me, but that effect soon wore off, and the cursing became a habit. I finally became ashamed of the habit, and struggled to break it. That struggle at least took my mind off my frustrations.

Then, in December 1978, my knees swelled up like a couple of balloons. It became necessary for us to test information we had obtained regarding veterans' benefits. Since my disability compensation was for damage to my back and lungs, we had doubts about getting help for rheumatism. But we need not have worried: At the Veterans Administration Center in White River Junction, Vermont, ninety miles south of Barton, I was classed as "service connected," and that seemed to be all that was necessary. I was entered into a large rheumatology clinic staffed with postdoctoral fellows, who were being trained under the head rheumatologist, Dr. Tom Taylor. I was given the latest anti-inflammatory drugs and received regular attention on scheduled visits.

That help came none too soon. The following month, February 1979, New England was seized in a cold snap, when for ten days the temperature on our hillside did not get above twenty below zero. Our water line froze, and we were running out of firewood. It was typical of me that at such a time I sought a solution to our crisis in my books. And it is also probably typical that I found the solution in a footnote in a combustion handbook. It said that certain woods, because of their combination of heat of combustion and moisture content, would burn fresh-cut, green; and ash is one such wood. We had a number of large white ashes near the house, and I soon became expert at cutting a tree to fall within a foot of a target. For the rest of that cold snap, I felled and split our large ash trees, and carted them through the snow to the waiting fires in our unfinished house.

From that spring on, things could only get better. Some people who had known me called to offer freelance work. I learned from my books to do the plumbing, electrical wiring, and carpentry work needed to finish our house. The regular scheduled visits to the rheumatology clinic at the VA hospital kept my rheumatism in check. Then, in 1985, I became eligible for Social Security, which afforded us just enough money to take the desperate edge off our economy. Dolly had a couple shows of her paintings, became represented by the Gallery 2, in Woodstock, Vermont, and even sold some paintings.

But everything collapsed for me in the winter of 1987. I had twisted my left knee while snowshoeing in the woods above our house. It was extremely painful, and with that, the rheumatism in that knee seemed to graduate into something different. Dr. Taylor diagnosed it as "pseudo gout," meaning that crystals of calcium and phosphorus were depositing in my knee joint, where they grated like grains of sand between the ends of my thighbone and shinbone as they rubbed against one another in the joint. The pain gave my visits to the rheumatology clinic a sense of desperation: It seemed essential that fluid be drained out of my knee and an injection of cortisone added every six weeks. As time went on, I needed that treatment more frequently. However, the rheumatology fellows had learned of the undesirable side effects of cortisone (steroid diabetes, muscle wasting, fatty face, loss of water, congestive heart failure, hirsutism, etc.), and they refused to shorten the interval between treatments.

Gradually, as my knee became more and more painful, I became more desperate. I found that no amount of will-power enabled me to put my full weight on that leg. I must have resembled a dope addict, as I avidly watched one rheumatology fellow after another first locate the spot beside my kneecap, then give an injection of painkiller, and finally push the large syringe two to three inches into my knee, until it reached the space under the kneecap. Then he or she would pull back the plunger, withdrawing fluid, until no more came out, and finally, replacing the tube attached to the syringe with another containing cortisone, carefully inject that tube of cortisone into my knee.

One day, one of the fellows whom I had been pressing for a more frequent treatment said, "I'm recommending you for a total knee," and he handed me a prescription form on which he had written simply "TK," meaning that my knee joint was to be replaced by a combination of plastic and stainless steel that had grown out of Frank Gunston's research. That prescription enrolled me in the VA hospital's orthopedic clinic, where the atmosphere was completely different from that in the rheumatology clinic. The familiar crew of rheumatology fellows was replaced by resident surgeons from the Dartmouth-Hitchcock Medical Center in Lebanon, New Hampshire, across the river. One immediately sensed that, whereas in the rheumatology clinic the action between the fellow and his or her patient took place in the small examining rooms, in the orthopedic clinic those examining rooms served only to plan for and review an action that took place elsewhere. I had grown used to the rheumatologists and felt ill at ease with the surgeons. Besides, I distrusted the very idea of an artificial knee, which brought to my mind the artificial legs that replace amputated legs.

Consequently, on my first interview with the staff surgeon, I told him that I would want no part of his artificial knee. He was quick to accept my decision, and he wrote out a prescription for a brace.

But the pain persisted. It was making an invalid of me, such that it would be impossible for Dolly and me to continue our life in Vermont. On increasingly frequent visits to the orthopedic clinic, I tried to change the direction of my treatment. I began to accept the idea that an artificial knee could be installed inside my leg to replace the deteriorated ends of my thighbone and shinbone in my knee joint. However, X-rays of my knee showed the bones to be in good condition relative to other patients. Because the operation was expensive, the VA tried to restrict its use. Although we had no insurance to cover my medical expenses, I had to consider engaging a surgeon, even if it meant selling our house. I got an estimate from the Dartmouth-Hitchcock Medical Center of some $15,000 for a total knee. As a possible alternative, I made an appointment to see Dr. James Maas, a much-respected surgeon in nearby Newport, Vermont. He described an arthroscopy as a "noninvasive" operation in which special fibers that carry sight around a turn, like liquid through pipe, are used to look inside a knee joint. The knee joint is pumped up with fluid and inspected by means of the fiber optics. Reaching in through a tube, the surgeon can snip off a piece of loose cartilage and perform other such minor operations. Dr. Maas said that such an operation would cost about $1,200, and he recommended that I have one before committing to a full knee replacement.

Dr. Maas's opinion seemed to be all that was necessary. On my next visit to the VA hospital, I asked the orthopedic resident about arthroscopy. He replied, "It might be a good idea to put a scope on you," and scheduled an arthroscopy. Two weeks later, I was on a mobile operating room bed, on my way to the operating room, when I again met the staff surgeon, this time wearing a green operating suit. He began reassuring me that this arthroscopy would enable us to avoid the total knee replacement, talking while the anesthesiologist was busy at my right arm. By this time I wanted that knee. I wanted to change his mind-set and was concentrating on what to say when his expression abruptly changed from friendly encouragement to regret and sympathy, and he was explaining that the surfaces in my joint were in such bad shape that nothing but a total knee would recover the use of that joint. They would be scheduling that operation for the near future.

I then realized that my anesthesia had been so effective that I had been put to sleep in the middle of a thought, had had the complete arthroscopy, and had wakened still in the middle of the same thought.

That arthroscopy occurred in January 1989, and it was March before the knee operation. I was lucky to have resident Dr. Mitchel Harris assigned from the Dartmouth-Hitchcock Medical Center to do it: X-rays of the knee he gave me have been used to illustrate an ideal example. It now functioned like a normal knee. My left leg was straighter. All my painful symptoms disappeared as if they had never existed.

And other aspects of our life seemed to reflect the condition of my knee. Although it was still not finished, our house was comfortable and attractive. Because we had learned what we did and did not like, we had a limited roster of desires. Through the many trips to White River Junction, we had learned to take advantage of the plays, movies, and concerts brought to the area by Dartmouth College in nearby Hanover. We had become familiar with Montreal, just ninety miles to our north. The Canadian radio had become a happy presence in our life. Most important, perhaps, was the confident independence that Dolly and I had won as a consequence of designing and building our house ourselves. Because we had consciously followed the principles in my engineering books and the tastes we'd acquired in Europe and New York, we liked everything and understood how it worked. We could fix everything ourselves, and the notion of outside help never occurred.

That brings us to the first week of May 1993, when it seemed that Dolly and I had survived a new crisis the previous winter. I had developed Parkinson's disease. Before it was diagnosed, the symptoms—an uncontrollable "stuttering" of my repetitive movements, such as brushing my teeth, chopping kindling, sweeping with a broom, or walking—kept me from even walking through our woods and was extremely frustrating. But by May, the disease had been diagnosed and I had entered a system of exercises and medications that promised to keep my Parkinson's in check. Always an optimist, I had begun to hope and make plans again. We little imagined, on Friday, May 7, as we cleaned out the ditches along our woods roads and raked leaves around the house, that I was to spend the next five and a half months without walking. Like so many of life's disasters, the one that overtook us then revealed itself only gradually.

It was still light and sunny at 6:00 P.M.—no more of winter's darkness at 4:30—when Dolly went in to prepare dinner. I put the rake away, but was reluctant to waste the wonderful daylight, and on the way in for my bath, I paused to give a turn to two pole jacks with which we were raising the southwest corner of our deck, where it extended from the house's first floor out into the canopy of the trees. As I tightened the second pole jack, the wrench slipped free. Off balance, I sought to step backward, but my right heel caught on the rough earth. With my Parkinson's fear of falling, I sought to sit down gently, but was too close to the edge, and found myself sitting in space. My feet appeared briefly against the blue sky, as the back of my neck bumped against an earth-covered boulder five feet below. My momentum carried me over into a backward somersault, and I felt myself falling helplessly, bouncing down, until I came to a stop on my shoulders, with my legs in the air and my feet behind my head. Carefully, achingly, I teetered over in a last controlled somersault to come to rest sitting with my right leg stretched out along the edge of a boulder at the base of the pile, some thirty feet below where I had been standing.

Frustrated and angry that I had damaged myself just when we could not afford it, my first reaction was to get back up to the house and pretend that this fall had not happened. Bracing my left hand on a boulder close beside me and easing my right hip off the boulder where I sat, I tried to lower myself to my left leg, which dangled down over the face of the boulder. But the left leg gave way, and I found myself hanging there by my hands with my right heel caught level with my head. At first, I couldn't lift my right hip back up to its seat. Pushing harder with my hands and right heel, I finally made it, and sat there, trembling, fearful that I had damaged Dr. Mitch Harris's knee.

Keeping my voice cheerful, I yoo-hooed for Dolly. She quickly climbed down, then back up to telephone the Barton ambulance, which arrived in less than fifteen minutes. With an inflatable splint on my left leg, three men carried me out in an aluminum tubelike stretcher, to a conventional stretcher and then to the ambulance. They took me to the emergency room of the North Country Hospital in nearby Newport, calling ahead, so that we arrived into a bustle of activity. They took X-rays and told me that I had broken my pelvis. I told them I was a disabled veteran and asked the doctor to telephone the VA hospital in White River Junction. When the doctor came back, they loaded me into the ambulance again, and we started south.

Meanwhile, Dolly had followed the ambulance to the North Country Hospital and had helped with the forms for my Medicare insurance. Now she followed the ambulance back south as far as our Barton exit, from where she watched its blinking light speed out of sight up the three-mile-long incline toward Sheffield Gap. Then she went back to our house in the woods to straighten up alone from the meal she had prepared but not shared. She kept herself too busy to reflect on what had happened. I had always taken a masculine pride in the self-reliance of our life in the woods, but it was she who now had to muster up the courage to keep that life going.

Next morning, when we saw each other at the VA hospital, I had just returned from a CT scan involving seventy X-ray shots, and she had taken a room in a motel across the road. She would stay there that night and the next, Sunday night, but she would have to return to Barton to take care of our house and would miss the first interview with the resident orthopedic surgeon. My CT scan had been ordered by another orthopedic surgeon, who had come in about midnight, on call from the Dartmouth-Hitchcock Medical Center in Lebanon. Encouraged by B. J. Ocker, the X-ray technician, who had come in that Saturday in order to have my CT scan ready for the surgeons to review Monday morning, we spent the weekend telling each other a prompt operation would fix my hip and estimating the days of recovery needed before I would be home again.

Only our ability to pay seemed to be anything to worry about, and I felt myself to be qualified both by my VA status and my Medicare insurance. Even after the experience with my knee, I was more concerned about losing precious summer time to work on our unfinished house than I was about my hip. Perhaps because I was unaware of what is involved, and because of the way friends and acquaintances had described their experiences of total-hip-replacement operations to me in terms of their successes, I thought only of getting a new ball-and-socket joint to replace the one damaged in my fall.

However, I spent the better part of a week chafing in my ignorance. Dr. Fuller, the chief orthopedic resident in charge of my case, did not materialize until the following Thursday, because he was attending a meeting in Boston. He presented the CT scan confirming that my pelvis was broken at a "fracture conference" held at Dartmouth-Hitchcock the following Monday, when it was decided that my pelvis should be given six to eight weeks to heal before a total hip replacement was attempted.

"You can stay here as long as you want," he told me cheerfully.

Meanwhile, the nurses had enrolled me with the Physical Therapy Department for a course of exercises and a walker. Knowing that the decision to leave was mine inspired me with a desire to leave as soon as I could—sooner than Dr. Fuller might have imagined. I disdained a wheelchair, but had to learn to use my walker with only a "touchdown" pressure by my left foot. The pain in my hip was something new. Encouraging us patients to avoid pain with codeine, the nurses would ask us to rate our pain on a scale of one to eleven. Allowing that the pain from a pinched sciatic nerve would rate eleven, I rated the pain that lurked just beyond my codeine pacification at seven to ten.

A major problem was the indignity associated with using the bedpan. Gary, a male nurse, finally resolved that problem for me by declaring in a loud voice that if he minded "wiping a patient's ass" or "cleaning up shit," he wouldn't be a nurse. I managed to time my needs to fit with his evening shift, 4:00 P.M. to 12:00 midnight. Finally, I felt ready to declare my independence and go home when, by using my walker and the chrome wall bars, I was able to support myself over the toilet in the bathroom in the corner of my hospital room. Dr. Fuller appeared gratifyingly surprised. However, the nurses objected and kept me there three days longer, until May 24, altogether eighteen days from that first Saturday.

The next two weeks were instructive. I had not realized the extent to which pain and physical disability sap one's moral strength. As always, I made the mistake of assuming good health right to the end. But the moment we arrived at our house, I realized that I was unable to climb the nine steps at the north end of our porch, and the only way for me to get in was backward, by sitting on each step, drawing my feet up to the step below, and then, with my hands gripping the edge of the next step at the small of my back, lifting and pushing to raise my buttocks. The pain of each part of that maneuver set the pattern for everything I would be trying to do.

Dolly desperately needed good nights of sleep, to re-cover from the exhaustion that overcame her during each day of caring for me. We learned the first night that I could not lie still in bed, so we rigged up systems of cushions on the sofa in our living room. Evening after evening, I determined not to bother her, no matter what, as I sought a different arrangement that would avoid the pain. But night after night, I found myself calling for her—worse, turning angry when she failed to hear me. My apologetic shame when she finally appeared, frightened and dis-traught with fatigue, only confused us both. Finally, we gave up trying and went back down to the outpatient de-partment of the VA center, where I appeared as a "drop-in." A sympathetic resident in general medicine had my hip X-rayed, then had me readmitted to the hospital. One more time, I was back in Two South, the surgical wing.

This time, we were prepared with a goal and plans based on experience. I resolved that I would be able to go home when I could (1) bathe myself and (2) achieve a full night's sleep. By now the nurses in Two South were all old friends whose help and advice I could count on. It was June 8, a month after my fall, and for some reason that wing of the hospital was passing through a slump in activity, with only fifteen of its thirty-six beds occupied. This meant that the nurses had more time than usual.

Also, this time I was alone in a four-bed ward in the western leg of the U formed by Two South, whereas I had previously been in a semiprivate room directly opposite the nurses' long counter, which extended along the eastern half of the bend in the U. The nurses' counter, their conference room, a kitchen, some supply rooms, and some bath and shower rooms equipped for bathing disabled patients occupied the inside of the Two South's U, with patients' rooms occupying the outside, where the windows were. Probably by design, those rooms facing the nurses' counter were either private or semiprivate rooms suitable for critical cases, while the rooms farther away in the western leg of the U were four-bed rooms. The operating suite with its intensive care unit was off the end of the western leg, and the elevators were off the end of the eastern leg.

With so few patients, there were extra wheelchairs standing in the halls of Two South. Also, there were several reclining chairs called "cardiac chairs" because they lifted an occupant's feet higher than the head when in the reclining position. One day soon after my arrival, a nurse, Jeannie, suggested I sit in an idle cardiac chair while she made up my bed. The chair was a relevation! The angle at which it held my thighs was just right, so that for the first time since my fall, I was comfortable enough to relax. Every night from then on, I would prowl the halls, using my walker, until I found a suitable cardiac chair, then climb into it and be immediately asleep, right there in the hospital corridor. Dolly and I decided we would have a cardiac chair the next time I went home.

That left my baths. Within a few days, Mary, a young nurse, showed me how to use the showers in the two special washrooms opposite my hospital room in the western leg of the U. She pushed me there in a wheelchair and gave me fresh towels, soap, a washcloth, and clean pajamas, then left me alone, on my promise that I would not try to walk without calling her. There was a chair with roller wheels that could be rolled into the shower stall. I learned how to undress, get into the roller chair, take a shower, dry, and dress myself before calling her. What luxury to be freshly showered and in fresh pajamas!

Within two weeks, I was able to take a shower by myself. The VA arranged to lend us a cardiac chair, and we were ready for me to go home. More important, I learned that an operation such as a total hip replacement is not to be purchased like vegetables in the supermarket or even a new car.

However, my newly learned patience was to be tested still more. On July 7, we got a letter from a newly assigned chief orthopedic resident, Dr. Geoffrey McCullen, telling us that he would be away on the day scheduled for my operation and scheduling the operation for a full month later. I wrote him, objecting; I asked to be scheduled to an earlier date, pointing out that the lack of exercise was making my leg muscles so weak that I would have trouble recovering from the operation.

Dolly and I went down to the VA center to discuss the possibilities. He was politely unmoved. I asked about having the operation done at Dartmouth-Hitchcock rather than the VA hospital; he said that might advance my schedule two or three weeks, but no more. (I reasoned that, with my Medicare insurance, going to Dartmouth-Hitchcock would cost me about $3,000, and didn't feel that a three-week advance in my schedule would be worth that much.) Finally, we settled for a program of exercises to get my right leg as strong as possible, and Dr. McCullen wrote out an order for the VA physical therapists.

The Physical Therapy Department at White River Junction was staffed by five young women—Charlene, Debbie, Jill, Judy, and Sue, who are perhaps the most popular people in the entire VA Medical Center. Their work should be depressing: They handle mostly men who are adapting to artificial limbs, recovering from strokes, or recovering from hip or knee replacements. The most depressing cases are the men with diabetes, who in successive operations have the ends of their limbs whittled away, toes, feet, lower legs, and so on, and who seem to be permanently enrolled in PT programs to adapt to their shrinking bodies. With those, as with all of us, the physical therapists maintain a restrained, professional level of sympathy and encouragement, which the individual patients desperately take personally.

Assuming that I knew, or could quickly learn, the principles underlying any exercise program, I had wanted to be enrolled with the PT Department simply in order to have my muscles monitored, and I expected to need only token visits, once the exercise program was outlined and explained. I was wrong on three counts: My muscles had already deteriorated more than I knew; the exercise program was more complex than I thought; and Jill, the physical therapist to whom I was assigned, assumed more responsibility for my recovery than I expected.

The adductor muscles in my left leg had atrophied. When muscles have deteriorated that much, it becomes impossible to build them up through direct exercises, because there are no muscles there to exercise. Rather, the exercise program attempts to build up related muscles, for example, building up my *ab*ductor muscles to strengthen my *ad*ductor muscles. The exercises used by the physical therapists are for the most part isometric, which means that you learn to tighten the muscles without moving. There were many times during the eventual hip replacement and recovery session when both the surgeon and the nurses sought and followed Jill's advice.

Meanwhile, the preparations for my October operation proceeded at a normal pace. The Red Cross notified me of an appointment to give two pints of blood, which would thus be on hand during the operation. And we made the trip to the VA Medical Center for a CT scan to be used by Dr. McCullen for planning. When I finally returned to Two South on October 20, the center was for me everything one could want from a hospital. I was assigned to a private room in the east leg of the U; and when I exclaimed about such luxury, the nurse, Pat, mumbled something about needing a particular sort of bed, which was then in that room.

At about this time, the field of joint replacement was being swept by the concept "periprosthetic osteolysis." *Peri-* = around the edges of; *prosthesis* = implant; *osteo-* = bone; *lysis* = dissolving. Reviews of the last thirty years of joint replacements had shown that the primary cause of loosening of joint implants was the dissolution of bone as the result of "macrophages," large cells that engulf foreign particles. Because the macrophages around a joint implant are unable to digest their ingested particles, which can be metal from the implant, cement from the implant-fixing cement, or polyethylene from the plastic, the macrophages synthesize cytokines and growth factors, parts of intricate cellular biochemical complexes that ultimately lead to the reabsorption of bone. While this bone resorption can be inhibited by indomethacin, an anti-inflammatory medicine used to control arthritis, the best approach to defeating this "particle disease" is through choice of material and surgical techniques.

Also, recent developments in tissue engineering were promising success in grafting articular cartilage onto joints. This material naturally occurs in joints and is almost magical in its slipperiness. However, it does not repair itself when it is damaged. This is at least partly because it has neither blood nor nerves. Tissue engineers are finding that an "osteochondral progenitor" cell, which occurs in bone marrow and the periosteum, may be successfully transplanted to replace damaged articular cartilage.

The operation on October 21 went according to schedule, with Dr. McCullen installing a total hip. Because of the condition of my pelvis, he cemented the polyethylene socket in place, with the extension for the ball of the joint press-fitted into my thighbone. I elected to have a spinal block for anesthesia, because that is supposed to have fewer side effects than a total anesthesia. I could hear Dr. McCullen's cheerful voice, over the sounds of hand tools being used, as though I were in a garage.

The day after the operation, I was sent to physical therapy to try to take my first steps in five and a half months between parallel bars. But I had lost more than the two pints of previously donated blood and was so weak that I hardly knew where I was and almost passed out. Jill, seeing how wobbly I was, sent me back to my room, where I received a transfusion. Altogether, it was seventeen days after my total hip arthroplasty (THA) before I was able to go home. During those days, I went to physical therapy morning and afternoon. Jill put me through exercise routines designed to get me walking. Both she and the nurses were careful to train me to avoid crossing my legs or bending so far as to pop my new hip joint out of its socket.

During this period, Dolly spent so much time with me that a visitor mistook her for one of the hospital staff. Later, Dolly told one nurse, Pat, "People think I work here." To which Pat responded: "You do."

Perhaps as the result of our living so long alone together in the woods, where survival required that we understand everything that happened to us, I was bothered by my lack of understanding of what had happened first with my knee and now with my hip. Since I had worked as an engineer and technical reporter, I had learned to study new subjects with producing a report in mind; and so I decided to write this book.

I told Dr. McCullen of my plan, and he offered to help with the book with as much time as he had available; I took him up on that to the extent that he agreed to become coauthor. On our way back to Barton, Dolly and I stopped at his temporary home, in Wilder, Vermont, and borrowed about forty pounds of his textbooks.

From here on, "we" means coauthors Geoffrey McCullen, M.D., and Ryle Miller.

We intend to help our readers cope with hip and knee problems suffered by themselves or their friends and loved ones. We hope to provide answers to the questions bothering Miller—questions we assume are bothering you or members of your family.

Hip and
Knee
Replacement

Chapter One

HARBINGERS of HIP
AND KNEE REPLACEMENT

WHEN MILLER EXPERIENCED a confusing lethargy and general aches during his vacation, he was right in line with statistics for rheumatism, which is defined as an inflammation of the muscles, ligaments, and tendons. Together with arthritis, which is defined as an inflammation of the joints, rheumatism attacks over 1% of all populations, usually beyond the age of forty. (Miller was forty-eight.) Women are affected two to three times as frequently as men. While the causes are generally unknown, the attacks are usually initiated by some form of physical or emotional stress. Thus Miller at first imagined he had strained himself carrying their luggage, which weighed in at ninety pounds at the airport. His sensations of unfamiliar sluggishness and early-afternoon fatigue are also symptomatic, and along with mental depression and stiffness in the morning, are said to occur in 96% of the cases of rheumatism and arthritis.

When Dr. Laufer had Miller admitted to New York University Hospital, he was being more efficient than Miller realized. Since bed rest is an effective anti-inflammation treatment, Miller was being treated at the same time as he was being examined. Also, Dr. Laufer was demonstrating sophistication when he insisted on calling Miller's ailment "polymyositis," meaning "inflamed muscles." Polymyositis is the description of a condition rather than the name of a disease; it thus has no implied treatments, whereas rheumatism, which also means inflamed muscles, has a number of recognized treatments but is classed as incurable.

Dr. Kantor displayed a matching sophistication by agreeing to hold off with his diagnosis, while treating Miller as if he had rheumatism, under the argument that Miller's reaction to accepted treatments for rheumatism would be diagnostic. Accordingly, Miller was entered at the NYU rheumatology clinic, where he was exposed to the gamut of treatments for rheumatism, including salicylates, hydroxychloroquine, indomethacin, cortisone pills and injections, withdrawal of joint fluid, and gold injections.

Injections of water-soluble gold compounds given with cortisone have been shown to be effective. Although gold brings on remission of the symptoms of rheumatism and arthritis, it can be of little benefit to patients with advanced arthritic joint destruction. And because of the risk of toxic side effects (dermatitis, albuminuria, hematuria, stomatitis, and other effects of heavy-metal poisoning), it cannot be given to anyone with liver or kidney disease; the recipient should have urinalyses and blood tests performed before each injection for the first few months of injections.

Gold shots are usually administered about fifty times at one-week intervals. Also, these medications do not change the natural history of the disease, so that when remission occurs (as happened with Miller) it is usually followed by a relapse after three to six months. However, the remission can be maintained by an administration of additional gold shots about once a month. Thus, although Miller does not appear to have realized it, he might have been able to change his lifetime medical history if he had been more patient and persisted with sustaining gold shots. We can learn the following lesson from this:

A treatment for rheumatism or arthritis should have continuity; and when you are required to move away from your doctor, you should be sure to find a new doctor who will take up your treatment in consultation with your previous doctor.

Although Miller seems to want to blame his pseudo gout on a twisted knee, his situation was that of the proverbial "accident waiting to happen," that is, his knee was in a state of sensitivity to any form of stress. As it was, the progression of his arthritis obeyed all the statistical predictions and explanations, as follows:

The bearing bones of our joints are normally protected with *articular cartilage,* a thin, tough, flexible, slippery surface, which is lubricated by *synovial fluid.* Like most lubricants, this synovial fluid is viscous and sticky. If a bit of healthy synovial fluid is put between a thumb and forefinger and they are spread apart, a thread of the synovial fluid will stretch out for as much as two inches between them. Synovial fluid and articular cartilage are one of the most slippery combinations, three times as slippery as skating on ice, four to ten times as slippery as metal on plastic (the Sir John Charnley joint), fifteen to twenty times as slippery as metal on metal when lubricated with synovial fluid, and more than thirty times as slippery as metal on metal lubricated with the best petroleum-based lubricants.

What this wonderful lubrication does for us is enable our joints to flex under pressure without wearing. However, over the course of time our joints are exposed to random extraordinary stresses, from the jolt experienced when missing one or two steps while running down stairs to the grating bend from catching a knee in a car door. As we grow older—and more of us are older, as the average age of our population grows older—the chance that our joints will be exposed to such random stresses increases almost to the level of certainty.

Whatever the stresses, the result is a deterioration that exhibits basically the same pattern. First, the articular cartilage is damaged, by crystals, as in Miller's pseudo gout, or by inflammation, as in rheumatoid arthritis, and bare bone surfaces are exposed to each other. The body tries to compensate with growths to alleviate the surface friction, but succeeds only in producing fibrocartilage and bone spurs. The fibrocartilage is not as effective as the articular cartilage, and the bone spurs can be broken off and driven through the remaining cartilage into the bone surface. The inflamed joint sends pain signals to the brain, inhibiting muscular reflexes, which leads the muscles to deteriorate and atrophy.

Although physicians insist that arthritis is incurable, a host of medical treatments, each geared more or less to a stage in this gradual deterioration, have become standard. In general, these treatments can be classified by function, as follows:

• Treatments to reduce the inflammation
• Aspiration of joint fluid to relieve pressure and run tests

• Treatments to repair damaged joint surfaces
• Replacement of part or all of the joint with artificial parts.

The last of these, joint replacement, has a higher success rate than the others. Consequently, you may, like Miller, feel impatient with the others, particularly when the rheumatology specialist caring for you insists that rheumatism and arthritis are incurable. You may share Miller's desire to bypass some phases of the progression and proceed directly to the joint-replacement operation. However, a total joint replacement is a major operation and should be treated with respect.

Reducing Inflammation

General inflammation and vague pain, such as experienced by Miller, are typically the first signs of prolonged, incurable diseases, like rheumatism and arthritis, that result from autoimmune phenomena. Contrary to what one might expect, the inflammation is not associated with an elevated temperature, although it does make one's skin feel warm to the touch. The experience is similar to feeling flushed. Typically, the pain Miller experienced was too imprecise to draw his attention to any specific point, like an aching thumb or shoulder. In fact, it took him several years to realize that the first sign of an attack was his irritability, as he encountered difficulty in performing familiar functions, such as putting on a sweater or tying a necktie. Because this type of pain is general and not specific, too many people ignore it. However, prompt, knowledgeable treatment can sometimes avoid, and almost always delay, the progressive deterioration that it forecasts. Moreover, the inflammation characterizing rheumatism and arthritis is not of itself as painful as the breakdown of joints and tissue that it causes.

The existence of inflammation can be reliably determined by a sedimentation test on one's blood. Called the erythrocyte sedimentation rate (ESR) test in medical terminology, this test is inexpensive, relatively fast, and easy. Sensitive but not specific, it can quickly tell the difference between a general inflammation that characterizes diseases such as rheumatism or arthritis and a local infection. Dr. Laufer appears to have performed this test himself, along with some others in his office. If you have seen a doctor because of an undefined pain, you would not be asking too much if you asked for the results of a sedimentation test.

Once rheumatism or arthritis has been indicated, you can count yourself in for a roster of treatments designed to reduce the inflammation. Although the purpose of these treatments is frequently described as the relief of pain, you will be making a childish mistake if you slight the treatment simply because you do not like to take pills and can stand that much pain. You should remember that because they reduce inflammation, these treatments inhibit its damage to your articular cartilage. Similarly, prescriptions for bed rest and splints or braces should be understood as anti-inflammation treatments. And don't let your doctor be upstaged by newspaper articles or hearsay, because his or her prescriptions for the early treatments of rheumatism involve commonly recognized procedures and medicines.

The list of medicines to reduce inflammation begins with aspirin. Again, because so many people think they know all about aspirin, we emphasize that your aspirin treatment is for the specific purpose of decreasing inflammation. Furthermore, when you take aspirin according to your doctor's prescribed treatment, you will find that you are not just popping a few pills into your mouth. For years, Miller regularly took prescribed quantities of ten to twenty tablets of aspirin per day, so that he constantly had a ringing in his ears like the hissing of an old-fashioned steam radiator, but McCullen says that no one gives this much aspirin any more.

The problem with aspirin, as with most of the anti-inflammation medicines, is that it is hard on your stomach. Again, if you are like many people new to these medicines, Miller included, you may take pride in your strong stomach. If so, rest assured that you will be needing all the strength your stomach can muster, in order to cope with medicines you will still be taking some twenty years from now. If you are presented with an alternative pill such as enteric coated aspirin that is easier on your stomach, choose that pill. The time will come when such a choice is not available. Then you should be sure to take some mild food along with the pill.

In addition to aspirin and the gold shots already mentioned, the list of generic medicines includes phenylbutazone, hydroxychloroquine, indomethacin, naproxen, and ibuprofen. Included with this list, but to be considered separately, are the corticosteroids, which are still the most effective anti-inflammatory medicine. There are about fifty varieties of corticosteroids. These medicines involve the adrenal and pituitary glands, which affect all organs and tissues by controlling the body's metabolism of water, electrolytes, carbohydrates, fat, and protein. The possibility that corticosteroids will take your body out of control, with consequent undesirable side effects, should limit their use to carefully monitored patients.

Aspiration of Joint Fluid and Cortisone Injection

An analysis of the synovial joint fluid is one of the most reliable ways to determine the state of a joint; it is the only way to confirm the existence of crystal-induced arthritis, such as pseudo gout. When combined with an injection of steroids, it becomes a treatment as well as a diagnostic technique. After the area has been anesthetized with a hypodermic injection, a large, 20-gauge syringe needle is pushed in between the bones of the joint to the space above the bearing surfaces, where the fluid collects, and then the fluid is withdrawn. Once the fluid has been withdrawn, the syringe used to remove fluid is also an effective means of putting corticosteroids directly at the place where they do the most good. The relatively easy injection has gradually been advanced in the roster of progressively difficult treatments, so you are now likely to be given this treatment for a swollen knee even before your first visit to a rheumatology specialist. Hip fluid is more difficult to aspirate, because the syringe needle must reach the space inside the hip joint. Consequently, you will probably have your hip aspirated by a rheumatologist or an orthopedic surgeon guided by X-rays. Because he did not find the specific "RF factors" indicating rheumatism, Dr. Kantor appears to have based much of his diagnosis of Miller's rheumatoid arthritis on an analysis of his joint fluids.

Arthroscopy

Arthroscopy is the application to joints of *endoscopy*, which is the general term for looking inside the body by means of fiber optics. Penetration to the point of observation by means of the fiber-optic tube can even follow a vein as far as the heart. Because there are typically no muscles severed, the technique avoids the trauma of much surgery. Consequently it has been extended beyond looking at an organ in order to tell its state to an expanding list of surgical procedures, such as removing cysts from the bladder (cystoscopy), removing tumors from the colon (colonoscopy), and removing bone spurs and even sewing together broken tendons in the knee (arthroscopy). Because the cost of a total knee replacement will be as much as twenty times that of an arthroscopy, arthroscopy should be considered first.

Replacing a Joint: Arthroplasty

Your condition could be such that your best available option is to have a total hip or knee replaced without further ado. In order to make the choice, however, you need to know just what is meant by a total hip replacement or a total knee replacement. *Arthroplasty* is defined as surgery to return the movement to the bones of a joint and restore the functions of the muscles controlling that joint.

ARTHROPLASTY OF THE HIP (THA)

Originally, the purpose of total hip arthroplasty (THA) was to provide surgical relief to arthritic patients over sixty-five years old who had been unable to find relief through the other means described above. However, the operation has been documented to be remarkably successful; and with some improvements, the technique has been expanded to include the disorders shown in Table 1 for younger, more active patients as well as those sixty-five and older with a sedentary lifestyle.

A total hip arthroplasty (THA) is a major operation involving a number of possible complications and an average
mortality rate of 1%. Because the hip cannot be isolated by
a tourniquet, as the knee can, there is a loss of two to three
pints of blood. Consequently anyone considering a THA
should anticipate the thorough examination given prior to
such surgery, in order to be sure he or she is not suffering
from unidentified ailments, such as a weak heart, low oxygen uptake by the lungs, hepatitis, urinary problems, hy-
pertension, unbalanced metabolism, diabetes, etc., that
would interfere with the success of the surgery. In addition, the nature of the THA requires that the patient be
free of certain specific disorders, including an infection that
could migrate to the hip joint, a disease that is destroying
the patient's bones, atrophied or otherwise insufficient
muscles, and a progressive neurologic disease.

A preoperative evaluation should therefore make sure,
first, that the patient is in good enough general condition
to stand the blood loss, both generally and from the hip.
Any anti-inflammatory and anticoagulant drugs should be
discontinued at least three weeks before surgery. Surface
wounds should be healed. Patients requiring transurethral
resection of the prostate should have that done before a
THA. If possible, the patient should give two or three pints
of blood a month before the THA, so as to have that blood
available for transfusion during the operation. Blood donations of one pint each should be spaced at least five days
apart. Iron supplements can be taken during the period
of donations.

ARTHROPLASTY OF THE KNEE (TKA)

The original purpose of the TKA was similar to that of the
THA, i.e., to relieve incapacitating pain in older patients

DISORDERS JUSTIFYING A TOTAL HIP ARTHROPLASTY

Arthritis
    Rheumatoid
    Ankylosing spondylitis
    Osteoarthritis
        Primary
        Secondary
Slipped capital femoral epiphysis
Congenital dislocation of hip
Coxa plana (Legg-Perthes disease)
Paget's disease
Traumatic dislocation
Fracture of the acetabulum
Hemophilia
Avascular necrosis
        After fracture or dislocation
        Idiopathic
        Slipped capital femoral epiphysis
        Cortisone-induced
        Hemoglobinopathies (sickle-cell disease)
        Caisson disease
        Renal disease
        Alcoholism
        Lupus
        Gaucher's disease
        Nonunion—femoral neck and trochanteric fractures
            with head involvement
Congenital subluxation or dislocation
Hip fusion and pseudarthrosis
Failed reconstruction
Osteotomy
Cup arthroplasty
Femoral head prosthesis
Girdlestone
Total hip replacement
Resurfacing arthroplasty
Bone tumor involving femur or acetabulum
Hereditary disorders

with sedentary lifestyles, or in younger patients with medical conditions that precluded strenuous physical activity. Because the design of knee prostheses has lagged ten to twelve years behind the design of the hip prostheses, the original applications of TKAs have not been expanded as have those of the THA. On the other hand, the knee joint, while requiring more exacting instrumentation, is more accessible than the hip joint, and the operation is less severe, without the associated trauma and loss of blood. The only patient disorders that absolutely bar consideration for a TKA are a current joint infection and atrophied joint nerves.

If you are a candidate for either a TKA or a THA, therefore, your specific case should be evaluated by your surgeon. Also, a preoperative evaluation should be performed by a physical therapist, who will oversee your rehabilitation after your operation. Typical physical therapist preoperative consultations for a TKA would get you started on quadriceps and straight leg-lifting exercises, as well as the passive leg-bending machine (CPM), which will probably be installed and operating before you are completely conscious.

Chapter Two

ArtHroplAst AnAtomy

THE MILLERS were enjoying a visit from their great-niece, Barbara, and her boyfriend, Jim. As they sat talking at lunch in the sunshine on their deck, Miller noticed the telltale faint red line of a scar running down the front of Barbara's knee and asked if that was the knee she had injured playing soccer. She yes, and he asked her what the operation had involved. "A ligament," she said evasively.

"Your cruciate ligament?" he asked.

She smiled, and proceeded to explain, while referring to her scars, that her surgeon had taken part of her hamstring tendon and used it to repair her anterior cruciate ligament. Jim then entered the discussion, saying he had two friends who had had the same operation as a consequence of football injuries. Barbara went on to explain that she was not typical of girls, in that her cruciate ligament had been damaged. Girls typically had problems with their collateral ligaments, because their wider hips tended to strain the collateral ligaments.

You can know what Barbara and the Millers were talking about and get a general idea of how your own hips and knees work from Fig. 1, which shows the bones of a normal right leg as seen from in front, and Fig. 2, which shows them from the rear.

Since your primary concern is probably with your own hips and knees, we suggest that you get in front of a full-length mirror and be sure each of the following descriptions corresponds to the reality of your own legs, including the location of pains or other sensations, by referring your exposed legs to Figs. 1 and 3. We'll start at the top, with your pelvis, which holds your insides above your legs. It also provides a seat for your spine, as well as the sockets, called the *acetabulae*, from which your legs swing. Because of all the flesh surrounding your pelvis, you cannot easily see it in the mirror, nor can you feel it, except for the two parts, called *ilia*, which stand out on either side of your abdomen. If you put your thumbs on the widest part of your hips and gouge them in, you may be able to locate your *greater trochanters* and relate them to Figs. 1 and 2. There are a lot of muscles and tendons connected to your greater trochanters, so you will be feeling those and not the bone. However, your greater trochanter is a prominent part of your *femur*, which is the biggest bone in your whole body.

Now, if you run your hand down the outside of your right leg until you get to just below and slightly to the rear of the outside of your knee, you can probably feel your *fibula*, where it nestles against the side of your *tibia*, which is your shinbone. Note in Fig. 2 how your fibula makes a lump below the knobby end of your femur. You may have

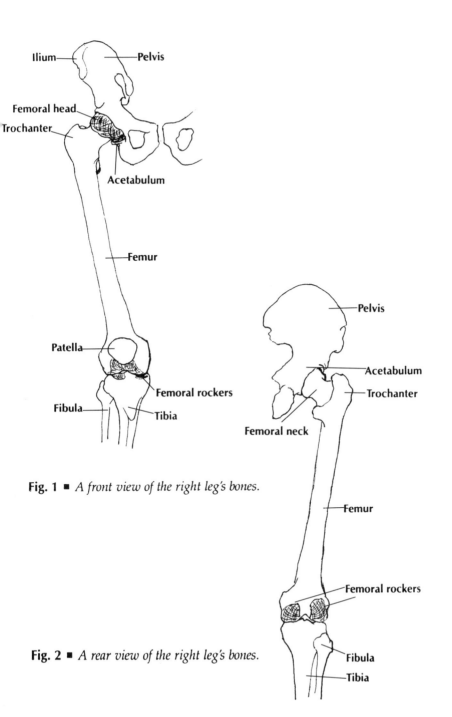

Fig. 1 ■ *A front view of the right leg's bones.*

Fig. 2 ■ *A rear view of the right leg's bones.*

some trouble feeling only your fibula, because of your *collateral ligaments,* which connect your femur to your fibula on the outside and to your tibia on the inside. They cross the area just described, but are not shown in Fig. 2. (Note: *Ligaments* connect bones to bones, whereas *tendons* connect bones to muscles.)

Putting your fingers on the front of your knee, you can probably make out your "kneecap," which is your *patella,* shown in Fig. 1.

Now, if you are curious about just where in your hip and knee joints you can find those remarkable but vulnerable bearing surfaces coated with articular cartilage and lubricated with synovial fluid, look first in Fig. 1 at the top of the femur, where the *femoral head* fits into the acetabulum. The rounded portion of the femoral head that makes sliding contact with the acetabulum is covered with articular cartilage. Then in Fig. 2, look at the bottom of the femur, where it ends in the knee. There are two shaded areas identified as *femoral rockers.* Those rockers are also covered with articular cartilage. Back in Fig. 1, you see a lopsided shaded area on the femur just below the patella. This area is that same articular cartilage, where the rockers come together in front.

The articular cartilage at that place covers a part of the femur called the *patellar groove.* The patella is attached both to the tibia, below it, with the *patellar ligament;* and to the *quadriceps,* the large muscles in the front of your thighs, above it, with the *patellar tendon.* Consequently you can use your quadriceps to step up by pulling through your patella to your tibia to straighten your leg. In order to do this your patella rides in its groove in the front of your femoral rockers.

You want to know why arthritic knees can be so painful?
While still watching your own knee in the mirror, make some ordinary movements (step up, turn, squat, etc.) and refer to Figs. 1 and 2 to see what your bones must do to accomplish those movements. You will see that your femoral rockers not only rock, but must also slide a little. Just imagine putting a pinch of sand, or crystals, underneath the femoral rockers, or imagine the articular cartilage diseased and shredded, and you will begin to understand arthritic pain.

More. Two additional pads of vulnerable cartilage, called the *menisci,* are also in your knee (Fig. 3): a *medial meniscus* under your inside femoral rocker and a *lateral meniscus* under your outside femoral rocker. The menisci act as shock absorbers between the bearing surfaces of the knee. It is easy to see that these cartilages can be damaged during stress, such as, for example, the pounding they get from jogging for an hour.

Fig. 4 shows what bioengineers have come up with to replace the bearing surfaces of the knee. It shows in X-rays of Miller's left knee an implant designed to accomplish the movements you can make. The total knee system comprises three principal parts: a tray and its support, which fit onto the top end of the tibia; a set of rockers, which fit onto the bottom end of a femur; and an insert. This insert is attached to the patella, between the rockers and the patella.

A closer look at the parts of Fig. 4 shows how their design lets them imitate the complicated movements of the human knee. The tray of Fig. 4 replaces the meniscal cartilages, so it is important to have the rockers in Fig. 4 contact the maximum surface on that tray, in order to distribute their loads. The rockers, viewed from the front, are wide, with

Fig. 3 ■ *A rear view of the right knee.*

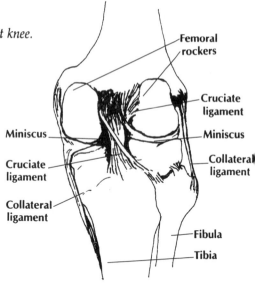

Fig. 4 ■ *X-rays of a left knee joint, showing the implants for a total knee arthroplasty, including a tibial tray supporting a tibial plate, plus a femoral rocker fitted onto the end of the femur and a patellar button (arrow) riding in the femural groove between the patella and the femoral rockers.*

Front view

Side view

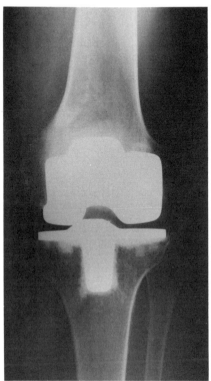

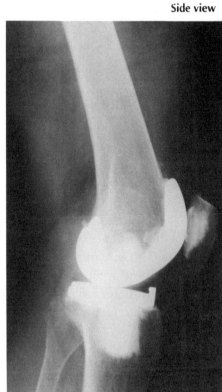

slightly curved shoulders, which gives a wide area of support while it lets the knee rock from side to side to a 3-degree angle. The solid metal portion between the rockers is grooved, like the femoral groove, so as to guide the polyethylene insert between it and the patella when one is standing erect. The inside shoulder of each of the rockers is also rounded, in order to continue to guide the patellar insert, when the rockers are toward the front of a bent knee. Between these two positions, there is a smooth transition from sides of the groove to the inside edges of the rockers at an angle of about 80 degrees, with the extremes being an angle of about minus 8 degrees, as when the knee is locked back, and about 115 degrees, as when sitting on one's heels. The tray replacing the meniscal cartilage has gently curving grooves with a 2mm and 3mm roll-back lip front and back.

The tray is made of ultrahigh-molecular-weight polyethylene (UHMWPE), which is a harder version of the same plastic used for coffee-can lids; its support is usually of titanium. The rockers are made of an alloy of chromium in cobalt. And the insert for the patella is made of UHMWPE.

Now let's turn our attention to the hip. We can use our new knowledge gained from studying Figs. 1 and 2 to surmise what happened to Miller's hip in his prologue, which is more than he was able to do. He says he somersaulted backward down over those boulders. This means that his femur was swung forward, so that his greater trochanter would be most prominent to the rear. After landing on his shoulders, he bounced from an outward-jutting rock, with the entire impact absorbed by the greater trochanter of his left femur, and the full weight of that impact was directed right into his acetabulum. The result, which is seen in Fig.

5, an X-ray taken after his fall, was that the femoral head was driven back toward the greater trochanter, while the receiver of all this impact energy, the acetabulum, was cracked and pushed out of its normal spherical shape (compare right and left hips in Fig. 5). Miller had difficulty lying on his back in bed or on a sofa because of the distortion

Fig. 5 ▪ *X-ray of right and left hip joints, showing damage due to a fall. Note that the acetabulum of the left hip (shown on the right side of the photo) is out of round (arrow), relative to the right hip; there is a crack in the left pelvis; and there is little or no bone to be reamed out for the acetabular cup.*

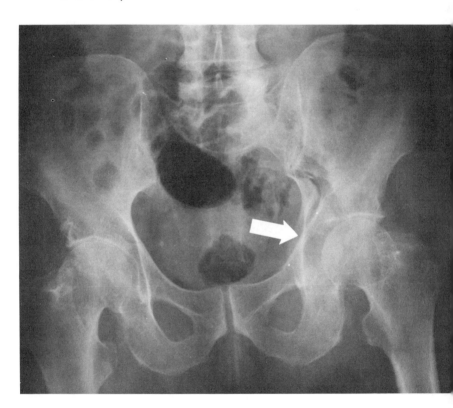

present in his acetabulum and his femur. The cardiac chair gave him relief because it bent his legs forward at his hips just enough to relieve that distortion.

The implant installed in Miller's left hip is shown in Fig. 6. One of the interesting things about this implant is the small size of its ball and socket compared to those of the

Fig. 6 ■ *X-ray of right and left hip joints, showing implants installed for arthroplasty to hip of Fig. 5. Note the cement required to compensate for damaged acetabulum of Fig. 5, and the small size of the implant's femoral head (arrow) relative to natural head.*

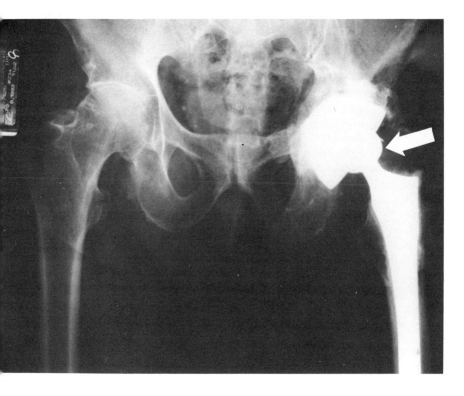

normal hip. This represents Sir John Charnley's basic development. Whereas it seems impossible to fabricate a joint
as well lubricated as our natural combination of articular
cartilage and synovial fluid, it is possible to fabricate a prosthesis of materials that are much stronger than natural
bone. Thus Sir John mounted a ball 22mm in diameter on a
slender stainless-steel neck, and the reduced bearing area
between the ball and the plastic socket correspondingly
reduced the frictional resistance to movement.

Since Sir John had installed some 10,000 of his hip designs by the time of his death in 1982, the collective experience with total hip replacements is statistically reliable for
durations of fifteen to twenty years, with both the problems
and their resolutions well documented. The duration of
Charnley implants was limited by wear of the UHMWPE.
Whereas increasing the ball's diameter reduced UHMWPE
wear, it was believed that the increased resistance to movement tended to loosen the cemented implant.

The adaptation of this metal-on-plastic bearing surface to
the knee lags behind the Charnley developments on the
hip by ten to twelve years, and there is not an equivalent
collective experience with the knee. Miller's knee, installed
in 1989, is still part of the statistical data currently under
development. This time lag is the result of the complexity
of the knee, which you have just confirmed by observing
your own knee in the mirror.

We hope that the preceding paragraphs have described
for you what is meant by a total joint replacement. Now we
intend to describe the THA and TKA operations and some
of the criteria used to design them.

Chapter Three

The THA and TKA Operations

B EFORE BRINGING A PATIENT to the operating room, a surgeon should make sure that the case has met four requirements: (1) a thorough understanding of the symptoms, causes, and background of the disease, (2) conscientious attempts to cure the condition through conservative, nonsurgical methods, (3) a review of the possible surgical alternatives to make sure that the selected surgery is the best treatment for the condition, and (4) a general medical assessment of the patient's ability to undergo the surgery.

You will probably have achieved the first two of these as you struggled with the underlying disease, particularly if that disease has been arthritis. Although you may not have looked on them as alternatives to surgery, you will probably have tried some of the nonsurgical cures, particularly

the anti-inflammation medicines. The alternatives to surgery likely to be attempted by a surgeon include a cane,
wedges worn in the heel of a shoe, specially designed
braces, weight loss, and a different pattern of activities.

When considering each of these alternatives, the surgeon
also has in mind such things as the amount and nature of
the inflammation, the state of the arthritis, and the specific
nature of the pain, as well as his personal evaluation of
each treatment according to his own experience with the
technique, particularly when the alternative is simpler
surgery.

Surgical Alternatives to Arthroplasty

The relations between so many alternatives are almost
too complex to be explained verbally, and the surgeon's
description may seem overly simple. Some of the surgical
"tricks of the trade" are described here: arthroscopy / debridement, chondroplasty, corrective osteotomy, unicompartmental arthroplasty, and arthrodesis. Each of
these is a surgical operation requiring an anesthetic.

ARTHROSCOPY / DEBRIDEMENT

Many people prefer arthroscopy to arthroplasty as the least
invasive operation, although arthroscopy is limited with
respect to a lasting cure. It is technically difficult to perform
on the hip and rarely if ever indicated for arthritis. It is
certainly a viable technique for removing pieces of tissue or
bone or bits of cartilage from the knee, as when the normally smooth, firm meniscus is torn or shredded.

Such a condition will be apparent during an arthroscopy,

when the surgeon may cut off the shredded end, in an operation called *debridement*, and correct the condition. However, an arthroscopy can provide a surgeon with little information beyond that provided by a sequence of properly done X-rays; and an arthroscopy / debridement may benefit only those who have a short history of joint problems, no problems with the alignment of their knee, and no degenerative changes shown in the history of their X-rays, but who do suffer from a joint that gives mechanical difficulty such as catching or locking or giving way unexpectedly.

CHONDROPLASTY

In some cases the articular cartilage may be missing, and it does not regenerate itself. However, a surgeon may be able to promote the growth of a substitute for the cartilage by drilling into the bone and causing blood to flow into the area not covered by the cartilage. The result is fibrocartilage, a cartilage-like substance mixed with fibrous material. While much less resilient than the natural cartilage, this fibrocartilage does offer some protection to the bare bone. Thus the technique, called *chondroplasty*, offers a stopgap remedy, but it does not preempt a subsequent TKA. It is suitable for people who weigh less than 200 pounds, are relatively inactive, and experience pain in a knee while at rest or at night.

Recent research into tissue engineering has indicated that there may be hope of regenerating articular cartilage. This ideal solution to resurfacing the bones of joints has thus far evaded us, because articular cartilage has no blood or nerves associated with it. However, two types of cell currently present in the bone marrow may be able to be grafted to the site of worn articular cartilage, analogously to a skin graft.

This means cutting and realigning a bone. Bad habits of posture or of daily activities frequently lead to *dysplasia*, or abnormal development. Dysplasia can also be congenital. Visualize the hip as a ball-and-socket joint (see Figs. 1, 2, and 6 in Chapter 2) and imagine that the femur, or thighbone, has been used so that excessive stress is applied to the leg from a given direction. The articular cartilage corresponding to that direction will get more than its share of the wear, so that it deteriorates. The body will signal the deterioration as pain, which will be associated with that position. This situation can commonly occur with machine operators, who apparently must either endure a life of pain or abandon their established means of livelihood.

However, a surgeon may intervene to effectively change the position, by cutting the bone and rotating it slightly, so that the habitual stress now occurs on different parts of the joint. Also the surgeon may be able to relieve such stresses by cutting away part of the joint and stabilizing the remaining bone with some sort of hardware either on the outside (in which case the metal supports are visibly fixed to pins through the skin) or on the inside (with the supports just under the skin).

An osteotomy is a viable alternative for relieving the stresses of a malalignment when the patient does not have other causes for joint malfunction. And when arthritis has produced an isolated area on one side only of a joint, and the patient is under sixty and not overweight, an osteotomy can be regarded as a temporizing surgery.

UNICOMPARTMENTAL ARTHROPLASTY

The knee has three working surfaces: the inside and out-side femoral rockers, each supported by its corresponding groove in the tibial tray, and the patella, tracking in its femoral groove. Unicompartmental arthroplasty means re-pairing only one of the rocker surfaces, in contrast to a TKA, in which all three surfaces are replaced. The opera-tion, which is technically more difficult for a surgeon, ap-pears to be regaining a popularity that it lost during the late 1980s. It enables one to retain both the anterior and posterior cruciate ligaments, as well as the other bone sur-faces; and the preservation of these joint segments is be-lieved to improve the ability to sense the limb's position in relation to the rest of the body—an ability important to many activities. The disadvantages of unicompartmental arthroplasty, which currently appear to outweigh its ad-vantages, relate to its operational difficulty: not only is it difficult to perform, it appears to make any subsequent total joint arthroplasty more difficult as well. In order to choose this option, the surgeon considers the alignment and the presence of any inflammation affecting the synov-ium, and thus the generation of synovial fluid. The tech-nique is suited to patients who are over sixty, engage in limited activity, have a good range of motion from 5 to 90 degrees, and have specifically limited joint damage.

ARTHRODESIS

Arthrodesis means the fusion of a joint. It is performed by removing the articular cartilage and using hardware to join the bared bone surfaces so that they can grow together. An arthrodesis may be advisable for a younger person who must be active to gain a livelihood, and who has a chronic infection that prohibits an arthroplasty on an extremely painful joint. But the joint no longer has motion, and this bone fusion may present difficulties to some activities, such as getting in and out of a car. Also, it puts stress on adjacent joints, and thus may lead to low-back or hip pains; and it is difficult, if not impossible, to reverse a fused joint and later install a THA or TKA. On the other hand, the procedure reliably eliminates pain and is durable.

Assuming that none of the surgical alternatives is appropriate and a total hip or knee arthroplasty is called for, the decision for surgery still depends on the patient's ability to pass the fourth test: suitable overall physical state. Thus the patient would be disqualified by a heart condition, sclerosis of the arteries, a malignant infection, diabetes, etc.

Procedure for the TKA and the THA

By far the most common and most popular treatments for arthritic hips and knees are the TKA and THA. These very successful techniques are indicated for otherwise healthy individuals who have failed to benefit from more conservative measures, are willing to undertake a significantly altered lifestyle, and have the ability and willingness to participate in a physical therapy program, which will be more than half the battle. Although the specific procedures differ, depending on whether the arthroplasty is of a hip or of a knee, the two operations share certain important features.

First, your surgeon, while flexible with respect to many aspects of the operation, will hold fiercely to a particular way of working, derived from his or her own personal experience. In the operating room, the surgeon will be backed up by a team of four or five people: an assisting surgeon, a scrub nurse, a circulating nurse, and the anesthesiologist and his or her assistant. The assisting surgeon, who has no specific function, is there to observe and help as necessary. The scrub nurse, who has a year's postgraduate training in operating room procedure, acts as the surgeon's immediate assistant, like a dentist's assistant, handing the surgeon the instruments according to hand signals. In many cases the scrub nurse will have worked with the surgeon so much that even the hand signals are unnecessary. The circulating nurse can act as a liaison between the sterilized and the nonsterilized environment.

As a patient, you will see most of the anesthesiologist, who is not only responsible for the anesthesia but also for monitoring your vital signs and caring for you during the operation. He or she will probably visit you in your hospital room both before and after the operation. Before the operation, the anesthesiologist will probably interview you in order to determine to a personal satisfaction your precise physical and mental state, including confirming such details as your blood type, allergies, and your preference for type of anesthesia.

The goal of the anesthesia is to put the area of your body under surgery into a complete coma, the effect of which is not only loss of sensation, but also loss of motor control. The difference between the different kinds of anesthesia is the area of the coma: your lower extremities only, or your whole body. With only your lower extremities involved, you have no control over your bowels or your bladder. With your whole body involved, your loss of control extends to your breathing. A "Foley catheter" is installed to drain your bladder during the operation, and the anesthesiologist must keep you breathing with an endotrachial tube into your lungs and a respirator.

The spinal block type of anesthesia is given in the lower back, either as an injection or as drops of the anesthetic fluid administered through a catheter. If you get a spinal anesthesia, you may be conscious enough to recognize from the following descriptions the various stages of the operation as they occur. Because of the tranquilizers given you by the anesthesiologist, you may find the experience interesting, even enjoyable, even though you are now repelled by the thought.

TOTAL KNEE ARTHROPLASTY (TKA)

The TKA is technically more complicated than the THA, but less traumatic. That is, it is more difficult for your surgeon but easier for you.

The knee is isolated from blood flow with a tourniquet resembling a large blood pressure cuff around the upper leg. (This represents an important difference between a knee and a hip arthroplasty.) The leg is sterilized by washing it with an antibiotic soap, then draped with a sterile cloth.

The surgery begins with an incision beginning three to four inches above your kneecap and extending down over the center of your kneecap for about eight inches, to the middle of the "tibial tubercle," the lump of tendon just below your kneecap. The incision is made quickly with a sharp knife, through the skin and the layer of fat just below the skin, to the underlying bursa (the small sack of serum between the tendon and the patella). The layer of skin and underlying fat can then be lifted clear of the sheath of membrane that lies next to the muscles, and the incision is carried deeper, down between the strands of the quadriceps muscles (past the patellar tendon), so that they can be spread apart. This frees the kneecap, or patella, which is flipped over to the side, exposing the knee joint.

The knee is now brought up from the straight position in which the incisions were made so that with the patella to one side, the knee bones project out through the incision and past the patella, where they can be inspected (see Figs. 1 and 2 in Chapter 2). The large front cruciate ligament is next cut free of the bone (see Fig. 3 in Chapter 2). With the femur so exposed, a hole is drilled into its end, exactly along the line of the bone, and the first of the all-important alignment instruments, a stiff support rod, is fitted into that hole. By means of this support rod, a cutting block is located at the end of the femur. The cutting block is then fastened to the end of the femur with screws or pins, and the rod is removed. The cutting block is then used to give the end of the femur a five-sided shape that will fit exactly into the femoral implant intended for your knee (see the "femoral rocker" in Fig. 4 in Chapter 2).

The tibia is next drawn forward on the freshly cut femur, so as to protect the blood vessels and nerves at the back of the knee. An alignment system consisting of braces and rods is fastened to the lower leg and used to position a cutting block at the end of the tibia. A saw is rested gently on the edge of this block, which is used as a planer to make a square cut across the end of the tibia.

Next, exact duplicates of the intended components are

used to make certain that all of these bone-shaping cuts are precise, and that the knee will function correctly with the selected components. The trial duplicates are sterilized and reused, while the selected components remain in their sterile packages until the surgeon is satisfied with the working of the knee.

A trial tibial component (the tray support in Fig. 4) is fastened to the tibia, and the polyethylene tray is snap-fitted to this trial component. The trial femoral component is put in place on that freshly cut five-sided end, and the knee is then brought into tension with the trial components in place, and exercised by straightening and bending, in order to see that it operates correctly. If the surgeon is not happy with these exercises, he corrects the surfaces, cutting off bony parts, and balances the tension on the collateral ligaments by using a scraper to push bone and cartilage up under them, so as to give them each the proper tension with the desired alignment.

When he is satisfied with the tibia and femur, the surgeon next shaves off the inner surface of the patella, either by hand or using a template clamp, in order to prepare it for the polyethylene patellar button to be cemented into place there. The trial components are then used to test the patella, tibia, and femur working in unison. The trial components are then removed and all of the knee, including the freshly cut bones, is flushed out thoroughly with saltwater solution.

The polymethyl methacrylate cement is prepared next. This is a "grout" (a filler that fits between two surfaces, binding them together) similar to the white cement used by dentists to fill cavities in your teeth. This cement heats up, as it polymerizes, to the point where it would be uncomfortable to hold a lump of it in your bare hand. The tibial component, patellar liner, and femoral component are taken from their sterile packages and cemented to the bones, which are prepared by means of grouting holes drilled into the bone. The knee is loaded and allowed time (about fifteen minutes) for the polymerizing cement to set. The cement expands slightly as it sets, so that excess must be chiseled away along the lines of attached surfaces.

The knee is again exercised to make sure its action is firm, and that the bones do not travel with respect to each other during bending. If the surgeon is satisfied, the tourniquet is removed and any sources of bleeding are identified and coagulated with a special electrical device. A drain tube leading out through the incision, so as to remove additional postoperative bleeding, is usually installed. The knee is thoroughly flushed with lots of saltwater solution, and the incision that separated the quadriceps muscles is sewn up.

The knee is again exercised, this time to make sure that the patella tracks properly in the femoral groove (a leading problem with knees). If the surgeon is satisfied with this last trial, the incisions through the skin and underlying fat are sewn up and a sterile bandage is applied.

Finally, the leg is put into a continuous passive motion (CPM) machine, which starts slowly moving your lower leg to straighten and bend the knee to about 40 degrees. At this point, which is about two hours after you first received your anesthetic, the operation is over. You are sent to postoperative intensive care, where you may be allowed visitors, before you are returned to your hospital room, where you will be in the direct care of the nurses and a physical therapist until you leave the hospital some five days to two weeks later.

TOTAL HIP ARTHROPLASTY (THA)

If you are to have a THA, you will most likely have been asked to give two pints of blood, with a one-week interval before the second pint, about a month before the operation. This blood will be waiting for you in the operating room to replace blood that you will almost surely lose during the operation.

On the operating table, you will be positioned, anesthetized, on your side opposite the hip to be replaced. The thigh and surrounding skin will be washed, sterilized, and draped similarly to the preparation for a knee.

Your surgeon will make an incision about eight inches long in the skin directly over your hip, and will carry this incision down through the underlying fat and sheath of fascia, or connective tissue, above the hip. As with the knee, these incisions are made parallel to and between the strands of muscle in order to minimize bleeding. Bleeding that does occur will be controlled by electrically cauterizing the blood vessels. Large claw retractors are used to hold the muscles out of the way on both sides of the incision.

With the femoral neck visible at the bottom of the incision, the assisting surgeon will reach in with a flat-bladed hook and, while your surgeon pushes down on your leg, carefully pull the femoral head free of its socket in the acetabulum and up. With the hip joint thus disconnected, your surgeon rotates your leg so that your knee is put over to the middle of the operating table, thus exposing the head of your femur.

The exposed femur and acetabulum are inspected to see if the articular cartilage and the bone surfaces are actually as predicted from the history of the disease and the X-rays.

If they are not in the expected condition, samples may be sent to the laboratory for analysis. If the condition of the joint is as expected, the surgeon prepares to install the implant, which will resemble that shown in Fig. 6 in Chapter 2.

This means that the whole end of the femur must be removed down to the greater trochanter (see Fig. 2 in Chapter 2), and the femur must be hollowed out to take the implant. First, the femoral neck is cut off, using templates to get the end of femur ready for hollowing out to fit a trial implant.

The acetabulum socket is prepared by reaming it out with a high-speed drill which is fitted on its end with a caged ball resembling a cheese grater. The articular cartilage is reamed out down to healthy bleeding bone underneath the cartilage. The surgeon is careful not to ream the bone of the socket so deep as to enter the pelvis. A trial acetabulum shell is press-fitted to the acetabulum. Normally this shell is installed for growth of the bone into the shell's porous surface, but Miller's pelvis was so damaged that McCullen had to cement his acetabulum shell to his pelvis.

Next, the trial components are used to exercise the joint the same as trial components were used to exercise the knee in the TKA operation. The surgeon manipulates the soft tissue in relation to the location of the lesser trochanter to obtain the proper length of the femur with its implant. This is not an exact procedure, and consequently the overall leg length may be changed slightly. Miller's left leg was lengthened three-quarters of an inch. When the surgeon is satisfied with the action of the joint, he or she cauterizes bleeding blood vessels and sews up the incisions.

Because the incisions have weakened the muscles that

hold the hip ball and socket together, there is always a danger that the hip may be dislocated right after a THA. Therefore, at the end of the operation, an "abduction pillow" is routinely placed between the patient's legs to prevent their being crossed. As with the TKA, the patient is sent to postoperative care, where he or she may be allowed visitors and receive a blood transfusion before being returned to the hospital room. The typical hospital stay, with daily visits to physical therapy, may be as short as four days or as long as two weeks. Following this period, the patient is sent home, with new crutches and a walker and instructions for exercise and care of the new hip.

Chapter Four

ANSWERS TO A $6 Billion QUESTION

H IP AND KNEE ARTHROPLASTY is one of the consistently
most successful procedures in all medicine, compet-
ing with coronary bypass surgery for the first place
in number of operations. In the United States in 1993, there
were 306,614 Medicare payments against $6 billion for total
hip, knee, and ankle replacement procedures. Total replacement surgery is almost never performed on ankles.
Allowing that the Medicare payments account for three-
quarters of the total number of operations and given that
surgeons do not normally work on weekends, these figures
correspond to over fifteen hundred operations per working
day, virtually all driven by the pain in a hip or knee. If you
get a new hip or knee implant on an average working day
four years later in 1996, you will probably be but one of

Table Two

HOSPITAL CHARGES FOR TOTAL HIP, KNEE, AND ANKLE PROCEDURES

YEAR	NUMBER OF DISCHARGES	TOTAL CHARGES ($ BILLIONS)	AVERAGE CHARGES, $	MEDICARE REIM- BURSEMENTS ($ BILLIONS)
1990	249,208	4.10	16,500	2.15
1991	278,631	4.85	17,400	2.48
1992	296,573	5.57	20,200	2.81
1993	306,614	6.03	20,600	3.16

Source: Health Care Financing Administration (HCFA), Bureau of Statistics and Data Management and Strategy

about 2,500 people who receive that surgery on the same day (Table 2).

There are many advantages in riding a wave of popularity to a medical treatment. Insurance policies will recognize the treatment. There will be many doctors familiar with the treatment, so that you can be assured of a reliable diagnosis and will be able to obtain a second opinion as necessary. Equipment will be proven and available. Surgical procedures will be well established. And the follow-up procedures will be worked out and available.

However, just because a medical treatment is popular doesn't mean it is going to be best for you. Any specific case may deviate from the norm, as is illustrated by Miller's initial experience with his hip. Although Dr. William Minsinger described his break in detail to him, Miller assumed, from association with simple broken bones, that a crack in his pelvis would repair easily; and from association with his successful TKA, he assumed that replacing his hip joint would be relatively easy. What he failed to appreciate was that a simple crack across his acetabulum rendered a THA impractical (Figs. 5 and 6). It was not until August 15, three months after his fall, that this was made clear to him, by Dr. McCullen.

Also, knowing that many people share your problem does little to relieve your suffering, and you are still likely to be at a loss about what to do. Even after you have consulted an orthopedic surgeon, have passed his or her "four hurdles" (understanding the disease, trying nonsurgical cures, review of surgical alternatives, and general medical assessment, as explained in Chapter 3), and have decided that you want a THA or TKA, the surgeon may suggest one of the many options (see Chapter 3). At that point the average cost of the approved Medicare procedures, about $22,000, makes your THA or TKA expensive enough to warrant a second opinion.

So you talk to a second surgeon. Then, assuming that the decision to replace the hip or knee is resolved, how confident can you be that the new hip or knee you get will perform as you hope? What will you want your surgeon to do about retaining your cruciate ligament in a new knee? Or about cementing or press-fitting the implant? And what does the surgeon expect to do about periprosthetic osteolysis?

Hospitals, the Key to Control

Although you and your surgeon share the direct responsibility for your new hip or knee, with a good half of the success depending on you (see Chapter 5), one of the approximately 4,000 U.S. hospitals will probably be the key to the success of your arthroplasty. There must be a good joint for you and your physical therapist to work with, and a good joint requires a well-designed implant with suitable tools for your surgeon to work with. Both the implant and the special tools for installing it will be furnished by the hospital. In 1993, hospitals charged an average of $20,600 for a hip or knee procedure, including $1,500 to $6,000 for the prosthesis, while operating room fees were around $15,000 for a knee and $10,000 for a hip, including the surgeon, the anesthesiologist, and the X-rays.

But the hospital's influence goes beyond considerations of cost. Your surgeon will be backed up by a specially trained operating team (see Chapter 3), who will be associated with the hospital. The specific implant the surgeon selects to replace your hip or knee (Figs. 4 and 6) will be selected from among at least three manufacturers and several dozen designs and sizes provided by each manufacturer. The instruments and tools the surgeon uses to install and test the implant will be of one specific design, so that even if your surgeon has evolved a set way of working to which he or she holds fiercely, the surgeon will need a stock of implants and instruments worth on the order of $500,000. These will be provided by the hospital, along with the operating room facilities, as well as the postoperative intensive care unit, the CPM machine, etc., etc.

Then there is a question of records. Although the X-rays are technically the property of the patient who pays for them, a series of X-rays taken from exactly the same position over a period of time is necessary to determine the progress of a joint both before and after the operation. Those X-rays should be maintained by the hospital. And because the science of joint replacement is still in a state of flux, every operation provides data for future surgeons, as long as all pertinent details of the operation are noted and recorded.

The equipment, personnel, controlled procedures, and storage facilities as well as the systems for recording, relating, and retrieving pertinent information for up to 3,000 procedures per day must come from the nation's hospitals, which are key elements in this mixture. Of the roughly 4,000 hospitals in the United States, some 245, or only 6%, are teaching hospitals, where resident doctors get advance training. Yet teaching hospitals account for 65% of transplants, including hip and knee implants, and for 50% of the nation's charity care. Furthermore, only a little over half of that number (126) are academic medical centers, yet the academic medical centers not only account for all U.S. doctors, they also perform 85% of the extramural, independently supported U.S. research.

The hospital will help you to review your financial position. Some sort of insurance seems a prerequisite, because the average cost of $22,000 is a heavy financial burden for people who are not wealthy. If you have Medicare Parts A and B, you will be concerned with the partitioning of the total average $22,000 into $9,000 to $19,000 for the hospital, $1,500 to $6,000 for the implant, and $6,500 for the operating fees and X-rays. The cost of your implant is included in your hospital cost, which is covered by Medicare Part A, and you are liable for only the fixed, Part A deductible of $716 (in 1995). If you have both Medicare Parts A and B, your Part B costs will come to $100 deductible plus 20% of your approved Part B costs.

The critical word here is "approved." Your approved costs for Part B are determined according to a payment schedule set forth in a "Diagnostic Related Grouping," a volume the size of the Manhattan telephone directory. If your surgeon has signed an agreement to become a Medicare participating doctor, he will abide by the Medicare schedule for his fees, and you will be charged 20% of the scheduled fee. If he does not accept the Medicare assigned fees, he can by law charge up to 115% of the scheduled fee, in which case your charges can be 20% of the scheduled fee plus his allowed excess, or 20% plus 15%, which equals 35% of the scheduled fee.

If you are one of the millions of Americans who are veterans of the uniformed services, you may be able to get your hip and knee problems cared for in one of the 120 VA Medical Centers located through out the United States. The VA recognizes, by law, two categories of veteran: (1) veterans who have service-connected disabilities, or were exposed to herbicides in Vietnam, or were exposed to atomic radiation, or have a condition from exposure in the Gulf War, or were prisoners of war, or are veterans of World War I, or have an income (in 1994) less than $19,912 if single with no dependents or less than $23,896 with one dependent; and (2) all other veterans who have an income (in 1994) above $19,912 if single with no dependents or above $23,896 with one dependent.

If you are in category 1, the VA considers you "mandatory"—the VA must provide you with hospital care at the nearest VA Medical Center, or if no VA facilities are available, in a Department of Defense hospital or other hospital affiliated with the VA. If you are in category 2, the VA considers you "discretionary"—you must pay the VA an amount equal to what you would have paid under Medicare.

So what does this mean? We think, based on the two points of view of surgeon and patient, it means that all American veterans have available truly superior hospital services. All but two or three of the 120 VA medical centers in the United States are associated with at least one of the 126 academic medical centers, with an exchange of residents and teaching doctors that assures the best-qualified care. Miller, for example, has had, in addition to his total knee and total hip, two life-saving surgical operations at the White River Junction VA Medical Center (one to remove a handball-sized abscess from his liver, and another to remove a ruptured and gangrenous gallbladder), plus years of treatment for arthritis, and currently diagnosis and treatment for Parkinson's disease. He affirms that, given the choice of hospitals in his experience, he would prefer the VA Medical Center at White River Junction.

If you have pain in a hip or knee and are a veteran, you are well advised to seek care at your nearest VA hospital. You can go, first, to the outpatient clinic, as a "drop-in." There you will be treated as part of a crowd, while you wait with a hundred or so other drop-ins. If you use your waiting time to observe, you will see an amazingly efficient computer-driven system at work. You will be logged in, with your identification being your name plus the last four digits of your Social Security number. Considering the number of people handled, your wait is remarkably short while a file is being created for you (or your file is retrieved). You are soon called to an interview with a nurse whose job is to decide which of several doctors on hand for the drop-ins should see you.

During this interview, you should bear in mind that the most important source of data that the nurse has to diagnose you is your description of what ails you. If you have already seen a doctor about your hip or knee, tell her. If you think that you have arthritis, tell her what you think and why you think it. If you are frightened by a dizzy spell that has just come over you as you were driving by, tell her that, and then watch the apparently chaotic drop-in clinic become purposefully efficient.

If you are there for the first time, the nurse will refer you to a patient representative, who will interview you in order to determine your category. Then you will see one of the doctors, possibly a specialist, who will enter you into one or another of the clinics, such as rheumatology, urology, orthopedics, or neurology. It may be that you have chosen to drop in on a day when the clinic for your ailment is closed, because its doctors are at the VA hospital or the affiliated teaching center. In that case, an appointment will be made for you to return to the clinic. When you do, you will be handled as you would be at other hospitals, except that you will not have the forms to fill out. Once your category is established at the VA, you are given a card, blue for category 2, or with a purple triangle for category 1. And all you need to do is to present your card, which is processed like a credit card.

Once you are being treated in one of the VA's clinics, its doctors will recommend you to another clinic, as they feel necessary. Thus we saw in the prologue how Miller was sent by a fellow in the rheumatology clinic to the orthopedic clinic. In fact, in Miller's experience, this method of referral is the only weakness in the VA system of clinics: The patient is sent from one specialist to another without ever being examined by a general internist. This puts the burden of responsibility on the patient to recognize and report any new symptoms.

All in all, Miller opines that the VA Medical Centers provide a current example of what would be available to the general public if we had a government-operated medical system. The most attractive part of the VA hospitals is their freedom from concerns about the "bottom line," a freedom that in our experience allows the hospital staff to concentrate on the patient.

What Happens When a New Hip or Knee Doesn't Work

Evelyn Zepf is a young woman with startling pale-green eyes who acts with a careful, quiet purposefulness that suggests that as a student she may have had to overcome antifeminine prejudice in pursuing her chosen profession, of mechanical engineering. Whether or not she ever experienced such prejudice, she now has a job that is completely without it—a job that could be the envy of almost any mechanical engineer, male or female. She is a project engineer in the Custom Products Department of Johnson and Johnson Orthopedics, where she designs one-of-a-kind hip and knee implants in cooperation with the surgeons who install the implants.

Her workplace is a small modern office with a drafting table and a computer. When we visited her, she had on her drafting table the life-size X-ray of a man's legs. One of the legs had the shaft of an implant sticking out through the side of the shinbone, as if the implant had broken through the side of the bone. She explained that the implant was still encased in bone, but the bone had grown that way in response to the constant imbalanced stress imposed over a period of years by the original total knee replacement. Most of Ms. Zepf's designs are what surgeons call "revisionist," which means that they replace implants that have failed. She showed us the template for her design to correct the leg in the X-ray.

We wondered about the availability of services like Ms. Zepf's as a source of reassurance to someone who might be considering a new hip or knee joint for the first time, and were told that Johnson and Johnson is typical of modern implant manufacturers in maintaining custom design departments. If we take Ms. Zepf's work as typical, the story of custom implant design is as follows.

Assume that some fifteen years after you get a TKA, you begin experiencing general intense pains in that leg. You go to your doctor, who refers you to a nearby medical center associated with a university. There you are referred to the center's orthopedic clinic, meaning that group of teaching and resident doctors plus students from the university's medical school who are specializing in bone surgery. At the clinic, you are exposed to the patient qualifying examinations, described in Chapter 3, including detailed X-rays. Then your case is presented, probably by one of the residents, to a "revision conference," in order to decide the best way to correct your leg. Depending only partly on the conclusions of the conference, one of the professors, who will be a senior surgeon, will decide on a protocol, and an operating procedure based on that protocol will be scheduled.

Assuming that a custom implant is needed for the selected protocol, a resident presents to the designated Custom Products Department (CPD) an inquiry, which would include X-rays, a description of the history and diagnosis of your ailment, and a general description of the implant needed for the scheduled operating procedure. Once this inquiry has been logged in at the CPD, the manager assigns a project engineer to that project. Then Ms. Zepf, if she is the assigned engineer, reviews the X-rays to make sure their scale is accurate and prepares templates for the designs proposed by the senior surgeon.

Photocopies of these templates are sent to the senior surgeon for his or her review and signature, and the signed photocopies, when received back at the CPD, become the surgeon's prescription order. Ms. Zepf uses them to prepare a complete engineering package of dimension drawings indicating the materials from which the implants are to be manufactured, the surface finishes, and any coatings. Also included are the method for combining the different parts (whether by press fit or other), and a set of specifications for procedures, quality control, and labeling information, etc. This engineering package is then reviewed and signed by one of her fellow project engineers at the CPD and sent to manufacturing engineering, where the manufacturing steps, along with all materials and required labor, are worked out. This manufacturing engineering package is the basis for a cost estimate for your corrective implant, and for a quote to the medical center.

This quote is the first you or anyone else knows how much your implant is going to cost.

Meanwhile, the engineering package is reviewed to see that the implant will conform to FDA requirements, as well as to quality performance criteria and the available manufacturing facilities.

If the hospital approves the quote, the implant is manufactured and shipped.

Trends in Bioengineering

Total hip and knee replacement procedures are now thirty years old, and they have brought entirely new concepts in bone surgery to prominence. The history of arthroplasty is in part a history of a marriage of medicine and engineering in bioengineering. The implants used in hip and knee replacements must take over the task of the original bone and last for many years, and they introduce problems in biomechanical stress well beyond those solved by the screws and plates that had long been used for fastening bones so that they grew together. Thus, for example, the pioneers in arthroplasty had to think for the first time about the mechanical leverage of a hip joint when a person stands on one leg. They discovered something sculptors have known since the time of the ancient Greeks—that because of the spread of the hips, standing on one foot while keeping the hips level exposes the supporting joint to roughly two and one-half times the body's weight. This can be worked out as a simple seesaw lever, according to the distance between the greater trochanter (where the muscles are attached) and the hip joint, relative to the distance between that joint and the centerline of the body (see Figs. 1 and 2 in Chapter 2). When activities like playing tennis are considered, the joint, or the implant, must be able to support up to twelve times the body's weight.

However, the stresses that the hip joint must withstand are slight compared to the stresses imposed by the range of motion that the knee joint must allow. Studies have shown that far from acting like a simple hinge or even a ball-and-socket joint, the knee joint passes during normal walking through at least four phases, including flexion, extension, adduction-abduction, and internal-external rotation, and that this walking action is simple compared to what happens in more complicated activities. Moreover, the desired stability of an artificial knee joint determines the type of implant as well as the surgical technique. Sideways stability depends on the collateral ligaments, the inside and outside meniscus, and the cruciate ligaments. Forward stability is provided by the anterior cruciate ligaments, rearward stability by the posterior cruciate ligaments, and rotational stability by various combinations of these. During normal walking joint surfaces are exposed to three times body weight, and during climbing stairs to four times body weight.

While it is not difficult for a mechanical engineer to design an implant to resist such stresses, the implant must also be designed for a long life, which introduces the concept of "fatigue stress." A metal will break when exposed to a sustainable stress again and again over a large number of times, or cycles. Also, our bodies with their salty blood provide a nearly ideal environment for corrosion. The key to solving these problems lies in the nature of metals.

Every pure solid metal is an element in the form of crystals. The strength of an alloy metal implant depends on the mixture of crystals it contains, as well as on the size and irregularity of its crystals. Smaller, irregular crystals make for greater strength. They are least deformed when the solid metal is cast into the form of the implant; they are made smaller and more irregular by heat treatment and forging or hammering the solid metal into a shape. Thus a cast pure metal usually exhibits minimum strength and forged metal alloys usually exhibit maximum strength.

The smallest unit of any element is an atom. By sharing

their electrons, adjacent atoms join together to form molecules, and when molecules dissolve in water, their atoms float apart to become ions, which have positive or negative charges, depending on whether the atom gained or lost an electron when forming the molecule. Because of their charge, ions will migrate through the water in which they are dissolved, when under an electromotive force, and such a solution is called an electrolyte. Blood is such a solution that contains electrolytes.

Because metallic elements like iron, chromium, and titanium form crystals directly without the intermediate formation of molecules, their atoms are packed together so closely that their electrons are not owned by any particular atom and are free to move through the mass of metal. This gives metals their common property of being conductors of electricity, and it also makes them susceptible to corrosion, which can happen anytime the metal is in contact with an electrolyte and is exposed to an electric charge. Avoiding corrosion is thus an important consideration in the design of implants.

How this is done usually depends on finding and breaking the weakest link in the four-step corrosion process. An atom in a metallic crystal gives up one or more electrons as payment for dissolving and becoming an ion, which is allowed to leave its crystalline home (step 1), usually from a tiny pit in the surface of the metal, and enter an electrolytic solution of ions in water, such as is formed by the salt dissolved in our blood. Then the metal ion must find transportation through the electrolytic solution (step 2), as its payment (the electrons) is transferred (step 3) through the metal's crystal lattice to a meeting place, only a micro-inch from the pit that it left, where the payment is reclaimed; the ion recovers its electrons (step 4) and is precipitated as an atom of metal again. By this process, the metal is transferred from a place where it is needed to a place where it is redundant.

Our blood not only helps this metal transport by providing the electrolytic solution to carry the ions in step **2,** but also helps in the desorption and adsorption steps **1** and **4.** Thus whenever a tiny electrical charge exists in or on the surface of an implant, tiny pits appear as bits of metal are carried off. One source for the electrical charge comes from the different atomic reactivities between metals. In this case the pits appear as bits of the more reactive metal, carried off in the order magnesium, chromium, iron, cobalt, nickel, and gold. Also, and more likely in hip and knee joints, the higher energy contained by stressed metal crystals leads them to act like more active metals.

Corrosion is avoided by interfering with one or more of the steps in the four-step corrosion process. Interfering with step **2** (changing the electrolytic solution) is ruled out because it would be hazardous to try to modify blood, and interfering with step **3** (changing the crystals) is ruled out because an essential part of any metal is its electrically conductive crystal lattice. That leaves steps **1** and **4.** Those steps of dissolving and precipitation can both be inhibited by coating the metal with some sort of film. Although an artificial film, like paint, is frequently used for corrosion inhibition in industrial applications, it would represent more foreign matter in a joint. Instead, implant designers have opted to select metals of which such a film is an inherent characteristic. Such metals are chromium, aluminum, titanium, zinc, and magnesium, all of which are so active that they react with oxygen in the blood to form a thin protective film of metal oxide on their surfaces. Among these, chromium and titanium are preferred for making implants because they are also strong. In fact, chromium is the basis of stainless steel, because 12% chromium alloyed in iron is enough to form the characteristic film. Titanium has the added advantage of forming a bond with living bone.

Today's total hip or total knee calls for bioengineering beyond the concept of reduced friction between plastic and steel, which Sir John Charnley originated.

The idea of a "candidate" for THA or TKA surgery as someone so old and feeble as to be unable to live long enough to exercise a pain-relieving implanted joint reflected the lack of confidence with which the early implants were regarded. However, the manufacturers of the implants rapidly improved their devices, as well as the tools used to install them. Those improvements, plus improved cementing techniques, brought about an era, in the 1980s, when people could be confident of pain relief for at least five years after the installation of a new hip or knee.

Still, the THAs and TKAs of the 1980s tended to loosen; and the possibility for expanding the roster of candidates to include younger, more active people led to research into the remarkable properties of bone to graft onto some metals, particularly titanium and metals with porous coatings and coatings of hydroxyapatite, a compound of phosphorus, calcium, and water with the same composition as bone. The resulting press-fitted implants produced excellent results in the hands of some surgeons. But as the practice entered its third decade in the 1990s, the long-term analysis of the results of thirty years of joint implants suggested that the use of cement had been wrongly blamed through a misinterpretation of the statistical data.

Partly because all of the early implants were cemented in place with polymethyl methacrylate dental cement, the cement was blamed for any loosening that occurred, and implant loosening was called "cement disease." However, these implants involved finger-packing the cement around a cast-metal implant with ridges and sharp corners. When improved techniques for pressurized cementing and well-designed superalloy implants evolved, the so-called cement disease disappeared. Instead, analyses of the data indicated that the loosening of an implant (the designs had been so much improved that a broken implant is almost unheard of) is due to particles of cement, plastic, or metal. In the confines at the edge of the implant, between the bone and the foreign material of the implant, the particles are ingested by macrophages, which are large mononuclear cells that normally engulf bacteria, digest them, and phago-cytose (break down) the digested cells into a harmless resi-due. However, the macrophages are not able to digest the foreign particles of cement, metal, or plastic that have been ingested, and the macrophages consequently release other cells that end up causing the bone to dissolve.

This hypothesized sequence of events depends on, first, wear of the articulating surfaces, particularly the polyethyl-ene, and second, an initiating crevice at the edge of the interface between the implant (prosthesis) and its seat, which can be the result of an automobile accident or of fifteen years of stress. The result is termed *periprosthetic osteolysis,* or dissolution of bone around the edge of implants. And the main cause of implant failure has come to be termed "particle disease."

The history of concepts of joint repair has thus moved through bioengineering to biochemistry.

Dealing with Doctors

We think of the doctor who, when a particular patient telephoned to say, "Doc, I'm dying," decided that the patient might not be feeling so well; but when another of his patients telephoned to say, "Doc, I don't feel so well," decided that that patient might be dying.

How would your doctor react if you told him, "Doc, I don't feel so well"? Or if you told him you were dying? Or how would you need to feel in order to tell a doctor that you didn't feel so well, or that you were dying?

We think that your doctor or your surgeon is like a singing coach whom you hire to help you bring out the best qualities in your voice, or like an architect who will work with you to arrive at a house that best suits your lifestyle and your property, or an investment counselor who will work with you to develop a portfolio of investments that best suits your circumstances and tax situation. Thus if you have pains in your hip or knee, you may hire a surgeon, who will work with you to develop a treatment best suited to the exact condition of your legs, and to your lifestyle. How much do you weigh? How old are you? Do you have arthritis? How do you earn your livelihood? What is the history of your joint problems? Do you have X-rays? And specifically what bothers you: Are you (1) under sixty? a participant in sports? without any previous problems? in trim physical condition? Can you describe your pain? Does your knee tend to give way, catch, or unexpectedly lock? Or are you (2) slight and relatively inactive, but experience pain in your hip at night? Or are you (3) a sixty-year-old skilled machinist who has begun to experience pain at work?

If (1), you could probably get some benefit from an arthroscopy-debridement; if (2) your surgeon might suggest a chondroplasty; and if (3) you might benefit from a corrective osteotomy (see Chapter 3). All of these treatments are minor surgery that, with the exception of osteotomy, can be performed in a "same day" clinic at most hospitals.

Our point here is that you should not either overstate or understate your symptoms to your doctor or your surgeon, but you should be responsible for a careful analysis of them. Don't be afraid to form an opinion about whatever ails you; and don't be afraid to read medical texts. The best place to discover a reference that applies to your specific subject is the current edition of *Books in Print,* which lists all the books currently in print, by subject and author, and should be available at most any library or good bookstore. Find a list of likely books, then try to browse those books at your local library or bookstore. Be sure to tell your doctor what you have been reading. He or she may have suggestions. You can measure your doctor's reaction against that of Miller's Dr. Laufer: one time, as Dr. Laufer was prescribing a treatment, speaking aloud to himself as he wrote it down, Miller blurted out:

"That treatment is right out of the *Merck Manual!*"

Dr. Laufer looked up, distracted, then grinned and said, "I'm glad."

If you try to hide the fact that you have been studying

medical texts, a good doctor will detect it anyway, because you will certainly give yourself away. More recently, Miller had an interview with Dr. Mary Luther, a neurology resident at the White River Junction VA Center. Miller, who had been frustrated by his symptoms, had decided that he was suffering from depression. He did not like the sound of Parkinson's disease, and wanted to argue when she made that diagnosis. (About the last thing a depressed person will do is to argue.) Whereupon Dr. Luther said:

"Look at your hands!"

They looked all right to Miller, until she said:

"They're hanging limp."

So he clenched his fists, holding his hands stiff, but she continued:

"And your eyes! You haven't blinked once, since you came in here!"

Miller was convinced.

This coin has two sides. By studying and actively participating in the logic of your treatment, you engage your doctor. If your doctor does not like being so engaged, he or she doesn't like practicing medicine. If your doctor assumes that you are not smart enough to understand medical texts, that is a strong indication that he or she also finds those texts difficult. In sum, by studying and trying to understand your medical symptoms, *with your doctor,* you are automatically screening your doctor for his or her sympathy toward you. If you find your present doctor does not pass the screening tests, you should find another doctor, even if you have already paid the present doctor considerable fees.

Another screening test for your doctor is to test him or her with a quote. Thus every new rheumatologist fellow, whom Miller was assigned to was told, "My old doctor called it polymyositis." The reaction was always clear-cut. Either a loud laugh suggesting that "my old doctor" was stupid, or a smile, with a comment to the effect that it had taken years for Dr. Taylor's diagnosis to be confirmed by crystals in my synovial fluid. You can decide which of those two reactions is the more sympathetic to you.

Chapter Five

LEARNING TO USE A NEW HIP OR NEW KNEE

Arthroplasty: an operation to return (1) motion to the bones of a joint and (2) control of the joint to the muscles, tendons, and soft tissue that surround it.

THE ABOVE DEFINITION is adopted from a textbook on orthopedic surgery. According to it, when a patient leaves the operating room, the THA or TKA is only half complete. The first part of an arthroplasty depends almost entirely on the surgeon, who has replaced nonworking bones with shiny new prostheses and tested them on the operating table for a working fit. The second part depends on the patient, who must learn to use the new joint, which will seem strange, precisely because the old joint was not working normally. Also, the leg in which a new knee is implanted will probably be straighter, and old pains will have disappeared. On the other hand, there will probably be a residual soreness as a consequence of the operation, and a new hip may change the length of a leg.

Immediately after your operation, you are sent to the hospital's postoperative care unit, where your heartbeat, blood circulation, blood pressure, temperature, and other vital signs are watched closely. You will regain consciousness there, if you have had a total anesthesia, or if you have had a spinal-block type of anesthesia, you will regain sensations and control over moving the parts of your lower body.

Taped to one of your arms will be an intravenous needle, an "IV," that enters a vein in your arm and connects via a tube to a bag of clear liquid suspended above your bed. That clear liquid will be a solution of ordinary salt in water, at the same concentration as the salt in your blood, plus vitamins and other food supplements. Also, your IV may be used to give you blood transfusions, blood thinner, antibiotics, and pain-relieving medicines—this last by your own command via a button you can push with your thumb.

You may be wearing special stockings that squeeze your legs every minute or so under air pressure. This is to keep the blood in your legs circulating so that it does not form clots, which could travel through your heart to your lungs ("a pulmonary embolism"). You will probably feel as if you need to go to the bathroom. If so, don't worry—that feeling comes from a Foley catheter, which is a tube inserted through your urinary tract to your bladder, so as to drain out your urine automatically to a bag hung on the side of your bed. Also, you may have running into your nose a tube, which has been feeding oxygen directly into your lungs.

All in all, you may feel that your body is merely another piece of equipment in the possession of the hospital. Again, don't worry: You will soon have complete control returned to you, probably before you feel quite ready for it.

As you become aware of your surroundings, you may be able to see that you are located in one of a gallery of beds that radiate outward from the center of the unit, like the chapels around the choir in a Gothic cathedral. And TKA recipients will become aware of still another device: the continuous passive motion (CPM) machine (Fig. 7), slowly bending and straightening the new knee from one to two times each minute. The CPM was installed on the leg with the new knee, in the operating room. Later you

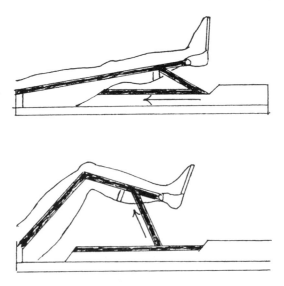

Fig. 7 ▪ *The continuous passive motion (CPM) machine exercises the knee to a given angle of bending.*

will be instructed to put your leg in the CPM machine, with your leg in its fleece-lined trough and your foot in its stirrup.

You may be allowed visitors in the postoperative care unit, and will thus have your first chance to tell others about your operation. If it has gone without incident, you will probably be transferred from the postoperative care unit before the end of the day. This is something you may want to note, because some supplementary insurance policies pay extra for every day spent in the intensive care unit. For example, the AARP supplementary cash insurance policy pays double its daily cash payment for days spent in intensive care.

If you think of a hospital as a place to rest, you can change that thought, at least for a THA or TKA. Once back in your hospital room you will be given one day to rest from the operation, with only your CPM machine going. Then you will be put to "work," doing things that may seem like hard manual work that you feel reluctant to do. You will be asked to keep the CPM machine exercising your leg for at least eight hours per day, during which you must lie flat on your back. Also, during each day, it will be necessary for you to be out of your bed visiting the physical therapy department, as well as to sit up and eat your meals, to wash, and to allow the nurse to make up your bed, so you will be pressed for time to put in on your CPM machine. Your nurses and physical therapists will keep after you, pushing you like straw bosses to greater efforts, because there is much for you to accomplish before you can go home.

The angle to which the CPM bends your knee will be daily increased by about 10 degrees, and you will probably be told that you will be free to go home when you have achieved 90 degrees. If you are like many others, you will become impatient with a daily increase of 10 degrees and ask for more; but if your physical therapist does increase your daily increment you will probably find that 10 degrees per day is about the limit beyond which the exercise becomes painful.

Before your operation, you should have had at least one meeting with your physical therapist, at which he or she will have outlined the program you are to follow after your THA or TKA. This meeting can be much more useful than a mere learning program. Just as the complexity of the interrelations between your diagnosis and the surgical possibilities made it difficult for your surgeon to tell you about his "tricks of the trade" (see Chapter 3), so also a physical therapist's attempt to describe for you the use of your new joint is often frustrated by the complexity of the relation between your past experience of that joint and the exercises through which you will learn to control the new joint.

Table 3, "What Hospital Patients Must Do for Rapid Rehabilitation of Hips and Knees," is based on a protocol prepared by Jill Cutting, physical therapist at the White River Junction VA Hospital, who was in charge of Miller for his THA. It shows the follow-up care provided by the hospital staff to the recipient of a new hip or knee during the seven to ten days spent in the hospital following the operation. The items on this list divide between, first, things to learn in order to adapt to your new body parts, and, second, the things you need to know and to practice in order to be independently mobile. Some of these things, such as "touch-down weight bearing" (TDWB), you will be able to forget. But you may have others with you for the rest of your life. The mechanical limitations of a knee implant, for example, may make it difficult for you to do things like ride a bicycle; and a slightly longer leg from a new hip may make it necessary for you to use a lift on one of your shoes.

In any event, the degree of success of the hospital's and the physical therapist's programs for your rehabilitation, as well as of your own home program for recovery, will depend on your attitude. No one can prescribe an attitude for you; you will develop one through following the hospital's program. Most important: Although you will be helped in just about everything you do while in the hospital, none of your activities, from the time you leave the operating room, should be passive except your use of the CPM machine. You must be an active participant in every part of the following program. We will describe the things in Jill's checklist; they are critical to the success of a THA or TKA.

PREOPERATION

During your preoperation meeting with the physical therapist, who will handle your rehabilitation, you should learn the purposes of the things you will be asked to do, including touch-down weight bearing, in which you use your operated leg to achieve the three-point gait (Fig. 8), and exercises, such as ankle pumps (Fig. 9), gluteal squeezes (Fig. 10), quad sets (Fig. 11), abductor-adductor range of motion exercises (Fig. 12), internal and external rotations (Fig. 13), and knee bends (Fig. 14).

One purpose of touch-down weight bearing is to enable you to use crutches safely. When you take your weight off your unoperated leg to move it forward, you will be

Table Three

WHAT HOSPITAL PATIENTS MUST DO FOR RAPID REHABILITATION OF HIPS AND KNEES

What must be learned

Preoperation:

    a. The overall purpose of the physical therapy program

    b. The purpose of touch-down weight bearing (TDWB) and the three-point gait with crutches

    c. The purpose of ankle pumps, gluteal sets, and quad sets

    d. The purpose of the continuous passive motion (CPM) machine (THAs excepted)

    e. Purpose of the THA precautions (TKAs excepted)

Postoperation:

Day 1

    a. Use of a wheelchair and a cardiac chair

    b. Use of the CPM machine (THAs excepted)

Day 2

    a. How to follow the THA precautions, including using the adductor pillow, getting in and out of bed, transferring from a wheelchair to a walker, sitting in a chair and in bed (TKAs excepted)

    b. Proper fit for crutches; three-point gait; feel of the touch-down weight bearing

Days 3–6

    a. Location, function, feel, and exercise of adductor-abductor muscles (TKAs excepted)

    b. How to go up and down stairs with crutches

    c. How to use a raised toilet seat (TKAs excepted)

Days 6–10

    a. Home exercise program

What must be performed postoperation

Day 2

    a. Begin walking between parallel bars, while observing TDWB

   b. Transfer from parallel bars to a walker and begin inde-
      pendent walking with the walker
   c. Perform ankle pumps, gluteal sets, and quad sets
   d. Practice avoiding unacceptable THA leg positions, us-
      ing a chair, a walker, a bed, and a pillow (TKAs ex-
      cepted)
Days 3–6
   a. Perform abductor-adductor exercises (TKAs excepted)
   b. Perform independent movement through corridors of
      hospital
   c. Use raised toilet seat (TKAs excepted) and perform
      bathroom functions of showering, washing, brushing
      teeth, and changing clothes
   d. Perform home exercises under therapist's supervision
   e. Advance angle on CPM machine to 90 degrees (THAs
      excepted)

supported only by your two crutches unless you put some
weight on your operated leg. You should put just enough
weight on your operated leg to stabilize your crutches,
while the balance of your weight is supported by your
hands on the grips. That way you maintain a three-point
gait—as you move forward, there is never a time when you
are precariously balanced on only the two points of your
crutches. "Touch-down weight bearing" means the maximum weight you are allowed for the operated leg while it
heals. (When Miller broke his pelvis, he was not able to put
any weight on his left foot. This meant he could not master
a three-point gait, and because he was unsteady with
crutches, Jill had him use a walker.)

   The length of your crutches should allow the cradles
about two finger-widths clearance below your armpits
when you are standing naturally straight with the crutches
at your sides and with your hands resting on the cross-
pieces, so that when you are walking with the crutches,

their full support goes to your hands, with no pressure into your armpits. Your two hands work with your bad leg and foot to maintain the three-point gait.

If you are tempted to imitate some unfortunate amputee who lives on crutches, and you want to swing speedily

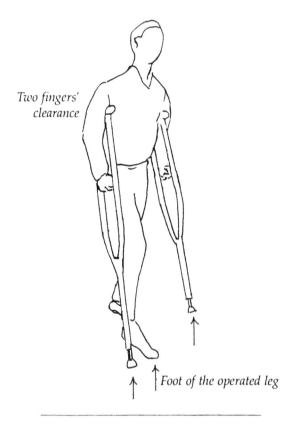

Two fingers' clearance

Foot of the operated leg

Fig. 8 ■ *The three-point gait consists of crutches (two points) plus the foot of the operated leg (one point) supporting the "touch-down weight," which is limited to 25% of body weight at three weeks post TKA, 50% at four weeks, 75% at five weeks, and full body weight at six weeks.*

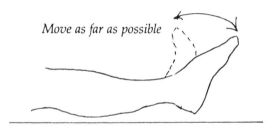

Move as far as possible

Fig. 9 ■ *Ankle pumps keep blood moving in the lower legs.*

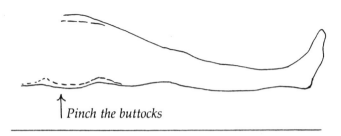

Pinch the buttocks

Fig. 10 ■ *Gluteal squeezes consist of tightening the buttocks; they are sometimes called "bringing up the squeeze."*

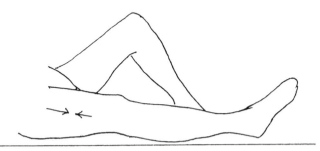

Tighten the thigh (quadriceps) muscle

Fig. 11 ■ *Quad sets tighten the muscles in the thigh to exercise those muscles after a THA or TKA.*

along with your operated leg dangling, remember the
adage "two hands for beginners," taught to young people
learning to catch a baseball, and think "three points for
beginners," for anyone learning to use crutches. Remember that your first purpose for using crutches is to exercise

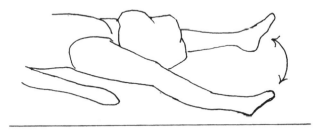

Fig. 12 ▪ *Abductor-adductor range-of-motion exercises help improve leg flexibility after a THA.*

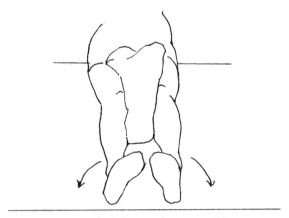

Rotate both legs as far as possible

Fig. 13 ▪ *Internal and external rotations improve freedom of movement after a THA.*

your operated leg; the three-point gait satisfies that purpose by allowing a controlled touch-down weight bearing, leading to a rapid recovery and a "two-point gait" by two healthy legs.

Also, you will get explanations of ankle pumps, gluteal squeezes, and quad sets as follows:

Ankle pumps are done merely by bending your ankles as far as possible in every direction (Fig. 9). Although such a simple exercise may seem to have little importance, this one could literally save your life. Ankle pumps keep blood circulating in your lower legs more effectively than the stockings and are every bit as useful in preventing blood clots in your lower legs as the blood-thinner medicines you will be receiving.

Gluteal squeezes are done by pinching together your buttocks (Fig. 10). This is another exercise that is deceptively simple relative to its importance. In Kripalu Yoga, over 30 percent of the exercises begin with "bringing up the squeeze," which is the same as gluteal sets. If you have

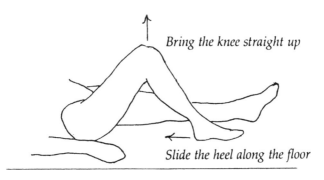

Bring the knee straight up

Slide the heel along the floor

Fig. 14 ■ *Knee bends strengthen muscles and improve flexibility after a THA.*

pains in your lower back, try "bringing up the squeeze" as you stand with your weight balanced on both feet.

Quad sets are done by tightening the quadriceps muscle of your thigh (Fig. 11). They are especially important after a TKA.

The precautions to follow after a THA are all designed to protect against dislocating the new joint. The two most dangerous positions are, first, bringing the thigh up forward to less than 90 degrees with the torso, as when sitting, and second, crossing the legs (Fig. 15). If you have had a THA, you will need to use raised seats to avoid bringing your thigh up too high as you relax into a sitting position, and you will need to sleep with a pillow between your legs to keep you from crossing them in your sleep. You should get the idea never to sit on anything low. This precaution becomes inconvenient when eating at a table, taking a bath, and using a toilet. It is important to have a comfortable, raised toilet seat, a tool for reaching down, and wall sup-

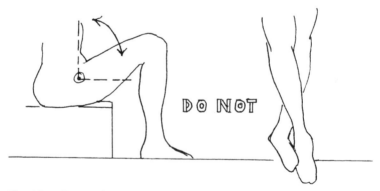

Fig. 15 ■ *Precautions to avoid dislocating a new hip joint include never crossing the legs and never bending to less than 90 degrees the angle between thighs and torso, for one month after a THA.*

ports near the toilet and your bathtub. You can console yourself with the knowledge that if you follow your exercise program, you will need to observe these restrictions for only a month. Also, this is likely to be one time when your physical therapist's advice might be followed over your surgeon's. The weakness associated with a THA is caused by muscle damage during the operation, and if your surgeon takes special pride in having minimized muscle damage, he or she may tend to downplay the importance of precautions.

Postoperation

The two principal goals of your hospital rehabilitation program are to get you used to the feel of your new hip or knee joint, and to prepare you for living with your new joint. In order to achieve these, you must learn to avoid damaging your new joint before its muscles have achieved the strength needed to control it. At the same time you will need to learn the feel of the joint through the exercises designed to strengthen its muscles. What follows describes both the precautions and the feelings you will need to learn, as you are put through the day-to-day rehabilitation schedule developed by Jill Cutting.

Day 1   Jill's protocol allows this first day as a day of relative rest when recovering from a THA or TKA. This means that the busy nurses will not have to occupy themselves with you, except to help you get into and out of your bed and a wheelchair or a "cardiac chair." A new THA or TKA patient's first introduction to the hospital staff will probably be with two specialists: a lab technician, who will wake you up on the morning of Day 1 to take some blood samples, apologetic about waking you and careful about the needle; and a nurse assigned to IV management, who, shortly after your blood has been sampled and still before breakfast or the appearance of the day nurse, will quietly come to the bedside, inspect the flow from the bag of clear liquid suspended above, then, leaning close, inspect your IV. On the first day "post op," the chances are that the IV nurse will nod approval and leave as quietly as he or she appeared. But there will come a morning before the end of the week when the nurse decides that the IV needs to be changed and asks if you would like it changed immediately or later in the day.

Alone again and awake, you may come to feel abandoned when no one appears for the following hour. But in fact you will be the subject of discussion at a regular morning meeting of the nurses of the night shift and the newly arrived nurses of the day shift, during which they go over the protocols to be followed for the various patients.

TKA patients will probably have the CPM machine constantly on the lower portion of their hospital bed, even when they are not using it. About the same length as a lower leg from foot to knee and not much wider, the CPM machine has a padded trough for your leg to lie in. The machine lifts the trough and inclines it at an angle under control of a small motor located under the trough. You can put your leg in it simply by lifting the leg over and lowering it into the groove. After the first day or so, the movement becomes soothing to the point where you may come to like and depend on it.

Day 2   Shortly after your IV has been checked, a nurse will appear and announce that you are scheduled for physical therapy at some time that morning. The nurse may suggest that you wash before going there, showing you where your washbasin, soap, washcloth, toothbrush, toothpaste, comb, and towels are stored in your bedside cabinet. The nurse will bring you a basin of hot water, but will encourage you to wash yourself. Washing in a hospital bed takes more time and effort than one might think, and you will be a little tired (and scarcely dried) when either your nurse or a volunteer hospital worker arrives with a wheelchair to whisk you away, speeding through the corridors and in and out of elevators to a remote part of the hospital building.

There you will discover that the physical therapy department is a bright room equipped like a physical fitness parlor, except for the addition of large workout tables that occupy nearly all the available space along the walls, each table being about two feet high, about the size of a bed, and covered with an exercise mat.

You will meet your assigned physical therapist, who will wheel you across the room to a set of parallel bars, and there you will begin the program that you were told about before your operation. On this first postoperation day, you will learn first how to transfer from a wheelchair to a walking support. With your wheelchair in between the ends of the parallel bars, you will be instructed to lift yourself to your feet while you support yourself almost entirely with your hands, firmly grasping the chair's arms (Fig. 16). (This will be the first time you have stood up with your new joint.) Then, standing on your good foot, you will transfer your handhold to the parallel bars. You will discover that your physical therapist has a webbed belt fastened around your waist and holds it as he or she walks along the bars and encourages you to walk between them, using the three-point gait, which you probably will have learned by the time you have walked back and forth a few times, supporting your weight with your hands on the bars as you touch the foot below your new joint to the floor.

Although mild, the exercise of walking back and forth between parallel bars will be tiring after even a TKA and a day of resting, so you probably will welcome the physical therapist's suggestion that you return to the wheelchair. But he or she will immediately push you over to one of the exercise tables and there begin to train you in the precautions you learned about in the THA preoperation indoctrination, moving your wheelchair to the exercise table

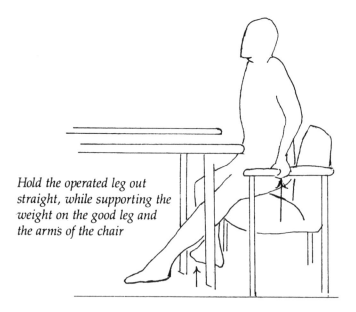

Hold the operated leg out
straight, while supporting the
weight on the good leg and
the arms of the chair

Fig. 16 ■ *Transferring from one support to another requires maintaining a firm handhold until the good leg is able to take the body weight.*

without either bending the operated leg to more than 90 degrees at the waist or crossing the legs (Fig. 15). The transfer to the table will involve a three-step maneuver: While keeping the operated leg straight, (1) rest that hip on the table about halfway down, then (2) slide the operated hip onto the table by pushing with the good leg, and finally, resting on an elbow, (3) move the rest of the body onto the bed (Fig. 17).

Once you are positioned on the exercise table, your phys-

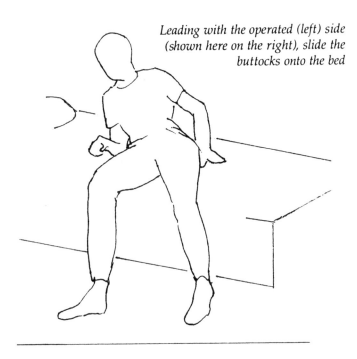

Leading with the operated (left) side (shown here on the right), slide the buttocks onto the bed

Fig. 17 ■ *The procedure for getting into and out of bed is one of the precautions to avoid dislocating a new hip joint.*

ical therapist will put you to work doing ankle pumps (Fig. 9), gluteal squeezes (Fig. 10), and quad sets (Fig. 11), until your legs begin to feel tired. By then the first scheduled time for the physical therapy program will be over, and another patient will be waiting for your physical therapist.

The nurse or volunteer will speed you through the corridors and back to your hospital room, which may already seem like a home from which you go out to work. You will find your room straightened up in your absence, the bed made up, your towels and washcloth replaced with fresh ones, and the curtains that isolate your bed from the others in the room pushed back to the wall. Your nurse will appear with a cart of equipment to get your "vital signs"—your blood pressure, heartbeat, temperature, and rate of breathing—and will enter them in your chart hanging on the foot of your bed. He or she will barely have finished when a person from the kitchen will appear with a tray holding your lunch. As the nurse leaves you to eat, while sitting on the edge of your bed, he or she will remind you that you have another appointment with physical therapy that afternoon.

When you appear for this second appointment, the physical therapist will take you immediately to the parallel bars again, but will not accompany you with the webbed belt as you make your trips back and forth. When you have completed several trips, you will discover that the physical therapist has taken away the wheelchair and replaced it with a walker. As you put your hands to it, he or she will ask if it feels right. It probably will, and as you look to see how it was adjusted, you will discover wrapped around one of its bars a piece of white tape with your name on it.

The walker will feel secure and easy to use, as your physical therapist has you walk about the room. He or she will tell you that you can take it with you and use it to walk around the hospital, if you promise to be careful. A promise readily given.

Then back to the exercise table. Miller first realized the extent to which Jill was monitoring his recovery when, as he was moving his leg in what he thought was the prescribed manner, she felt it and told him that his abductor muscle was not functioning. Alerted to the lack of sensation, Miller tried to make the movement but failed. The experience, while not painful, was unpleasant. It is not typical of THAs, and was a result of his fall.

Although you may have looked forward to using the new walker to explore the hospital wings and corridors, once released from "PT" you will have no time for such expeditions that day. Instead, your nurse will ask you if you would like to take a walk with him or her. When you return to your room from that walk, you will discover that the IV tower with its tangle of tubes is gone from your bedside.

Days 3–6 The morning of the following postoperative day, Day 3, the physical therapist will introduce (for TKAs) the knee range-of-motion and hamstring-pull exercises. The knee range-of-motion exercise (Fig. 18) consists of sitting on the edge of the exercise table with the operated leg hanging down, pulling that leg back as far as possible and holding it there for a count of five, and then straightening it out as much as possible and holding it straight for a count of five. The hamstring pull (Fig. 19) consists of lying face-down and pulling the operated leg up as far as possible for a count of five. Similarly, THAs practice the abduction-adduction range-of-motion exercise (Fig. 12) and the internal-external rotation exercise (Fig. 13). Both TKAs and THAs do the short-arc quads, which resemble the quad sets but with a rolled-up towel or similar object under the knee (Fig. 20), so as to require the quadriceps muscle to work a little harder.

Also during this period, the physical therapist will have you do things leading toward "functional mobility" (transfers between exercise table, walker, and wheelchair, as well as the touch-down weight-bearing gait with a walker) to the point where you become independently mobile in the hospital. At the same time, if you have had a THA, the nurses will help you learn to use a raised toilet seat in the toilet room off your hospital room, as well as how to use a special shower room in your hospital wing. Around post-operative Day 5, the physical therapists will begin your exercises in the use of crutches.

Your physical therapist will have you use only one crutch on stairs, while holding to a railing; and because of the danger in going up and down stairs with crutches, he or she will put the webbed belt around your waist and hold onto it as you first try. To avoid tripping and pole-vaulting down the stairs, you must always reach down, first, to the next-lower step with one crutch. That means you must support your whole weight, balancing, on your good foot, then balance your weight on one crutch and the railing with touch-down weight-bearing on your operated leg, as you bring your good foot down to the level of your crutch, and no farther. If you have a tendency to disdain the conservative three-point gait in order to move faster with your crutches, swinging along in a leapfrogging two-point-then-one-foot gait, never try going downstairs that way—your crutches would catapult you into space. Stairs can quickly

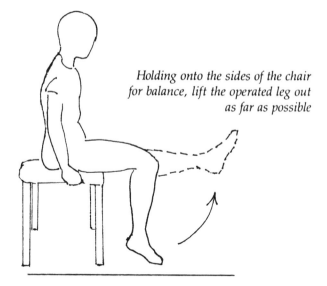

Holding onto the sides of the chair for balance, lift the operated leg out as far as possible

Fig. 18 ▪ *Bending and straightening the leg strengthens the knee and increases its range of motion after a TKA.*

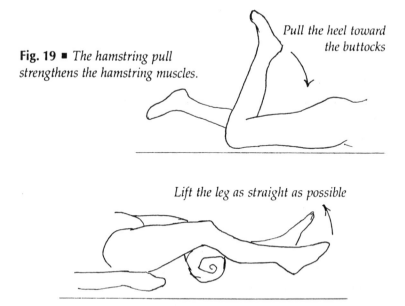

Fig. 19 ▪ *The hamstring pull strengthens the hamstring muscles.*

Pull the heel toward the buttocks

Lift the leg as straight as possible

Fig. 20 ▪ *The short-arc quad exercise is like the simple quad sets shown in Fig. 11, but a towel or other object is placed under the knee to impose more stress.*

teach you the mechanics of walking with crutches, including the need for clearance between the crutch rockers and your armpits, the role of your touch-down bearing weight, and the importance of the three-point gait.

You may still be looking forward to using your new walker to explore the hospital, but again you will find little time for such expeditions. When you return to your room from PT, your nurse will ask you if you would like to take a shower—a prospect too appealing to even hesitate at. But by the time you have returned, clean and with fresh pajamas, you will find that your midday meal is already waiting for you on your bedside tray. And by the time you have eaten, it will be time to go down to PT for your afternoon session. You may ask if you can go there on your own, but will be told that it would take too long, and you would be late for your appointment.

Days 6–10   In order to reduce costs, most hospitals try to get their THAs and TKAs out as soon as possible, while putting more emphasis on follow-up services after the patient returns home. This means discharge on the sixth to the eighth day after the operation for TKAs and only a day or two more for THAs. It also means that your physical therapist must train you in everything necessary before Day 6. And since THAs are supposed to avoid crossing their legs or bending to more than 90 degrees for a month after their arthroplasty, their training in some of the essential exercises must be limited until after they have returned home. We are including, with permission, sets of instructions for home exercise programs, which have been prepared by the Physical Therapy Department of the VA Medical Center at White River Junction, Vermont.

A few days in a hospital will usually make the notion of "home" seem like a safe harbor where the wounded and battered body can be brought to dry dock for leisurely repairs. A patient tends to overlook the fact that his or her home is also a safe haven for a number of other members of the family, who have come to look on him or her as reliable. Whereas you may be counting on them to do things for you, they may be counting on you to mediate, advise, and help, as you have conditioned them to count on you in the past.

A first shock will probably come from your wishful thinking that annoying aspects of your new hip or knee will disappear once you are on your familiar home territory. A new hip may have made your leg up to an inch longer, and a new knee may be mechanically limited in the amount you can bend it. Although you may have tried to overlook such problems in the hospital, they will become continuing annoyances at home. You will need to exercise the new knee. The difference in leg lengths must be compensated for with shoe modifications or it may lead to chronic back pains.

After considerable experimenting, Miller found that the best compensation was a thicker heel and sole in the shoe of the shorter leg, with more compensation in the heel than in the sole. In general terms, he found that the difference can be determined either by the surgeon from X-rays or by a physical therapist, who fits different thicknesses of felt or rubber under the sole of the shorter leg until the hips are level. He found that for general moving and walking, the most comfortable adaptation consisted of a gradually sloping lift, from about 110% of the difference in leg length at the rear of his heel to about 25% of that difference at the front of his foot, with 75% of the difference at the ball of his foot and the exact 100% difference only at the front of his heel. And he found that the most comfortable shoe was a sneaker (Fig. 21). While a lift with a single thickness seemed comfortable when he was standing still, it became awkward when he began to move.

Also, you must give some thought and care to infection. Because the implant materials of arthroplasties are foreign to the fluids and tissues of the body, they appear to attract some infections. And many hospitals provide the discharged THA or TKA with a prescription for antibiotic medicine to be taken when having dental work done.

Other things to provide for a safe and comfortable rehabilitation at home include handrails for a shower, pain pills, a seat for the bathtub, a two-foot-long grasping tool, and a raised seat for the toilet. The handrails are likely to be used more and more as you become habituated to them, whereas the other things are likely to become unnecessary as you get more familiar with your new joint.

The most important thing to take home with you will

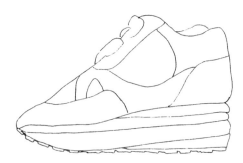

Fig. 21 ▪ *A sneaker with a built-up sole has proved to be the best compensation for Miller's lengthened leg.*

be your attitude, bolstered by habits acquired during your sessions of physical training, plus a set of exercises to do at home. Your attitude should be that of a creative painter or sculptor, working with your body to make something out of it. Although you may hope to achieve given things, such as swimming, or hiking a remembered trail, nothing can be taken for granted, and you will necessarily modify your ambitions as you daily discover what your body is and is not able to do.

Accordingly, your exercises, in addition to training your muscles, will serve as a guide by which you must adjust your ultimate goals. For example, the schedule by which you increase the fraction of your total body weight carried by your operated leg, increasing 25% for each additional week after three weeks postoperation, can be a target and a guide, so that at seven weeks after your operation, you can begin walking with only one crutch in the hand opposite your operated leg. Similarly, the range-of-motion exercises can set the pace for a THA's recovery. Of all the home exercises, walking is perhaps the best criterion of improvement. You should walk several times each day, and you should make note of how far and how easily you walked.

Unfortunately, most of your exercises are not measured according to distance, like walking, or according to weight supported, like the TDWB. Yet these exercises are essential to your rehabilitation, and their effects can be measured in terms of the others. For example, it would be a mistake to assume that because distance walked is measurable, you could abandon all other exercises in order to concentrate on walking.

Foremost among the exercises are those designed to strengthen your stomach and back muscles. Do these each day, and see how easy it becomes for you to do other things. The strengthening exercises are the knee-to-chest stretch, the hip-rotator stretch, the abdominal lift, and the partial curl-up. These four exercises can be done in no more than half an hour, they are easy to do, and if they are practiced in a daily routine they will keep you looking and feeling trim.

The knee-to-chest stretch (Fig. 22) comes as a natural sequel to the knee bends (Fig. 14), after one month during which your hip muscles have become strong enough so

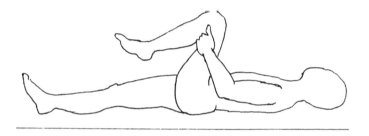

Fig. 22 ▪ *The knee-to-chest stretch extends the knee-bending exercise.*

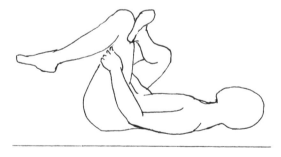

Fig. 23 ▪ *The hip-rotator stretch flexes the hip muscles.*

that you no longer must observe the THA precautions (Fig. 15). It stretches the muscles in the lower back, in addition to strengthening the abductor-adductor muscles. While lying on your back with one leg bent, grasp the thigh behind your bent leg and pull the thigh to your chest. Hold for a count of 20 (20 seconds) and release.

The hip-rotator stretch (Fig. 23) comes as a natural sequel to the knee-to-chest stretch. While lying flat on your back with one leg bent, cross your legs so that the ankle of one leg rests against the thigh of the other leg. Then grasp your bent leg behind the thigh and pull that leg toward your

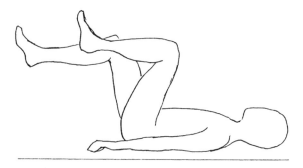

Fig. 24 ▪ *The abdominal lift strengthens the lower abdomen and hip muscles.*

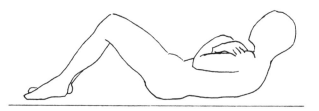

Fig. 25 ▪ *The partial curl-up strengthens the upper abdomen.*

chest. This exercise will enable you to squat and cross your legs more easily.

The abdominal lift (Fig. 24) strengthens the muscles of your lower abdomen and balances the strengths of the muscles around your hips. While lying on your back with both legs bent, lift first one leg, then the other, and with both legs in the air alternately straighten and bend them, like bicycling, except for keeping your shinbones parallel to the floor. Do this for 20 seconds.

The partial curl-up (Fig. 25) is a well-known and popular exercise for strengthening the stomach muscles. While lying on your back with both legs drawn up and your wrists crossed on your chest, lift your shoulder blades off the floor up to an angle of only 30 degrees. Hold for 5 seconds and repeat.

Index

Page numbers in *italics* refer to illustrations and tables.

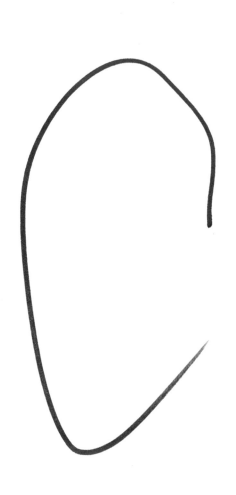